# Concept Mapping:

## A Critical-Thinking Approach to Care Planning

# Concept Mapping:

## A CRITICAL-THINKING APPROACH TO CARE PLANNING

**Pamela McHugh Schuster,** RN, PhD

Professor of Nursing
Youngstown State University
Youngstown, Ohio

F.A. Davis Company / Philadelphia

F. A. Davis Company
1915 Arch Street
Philadelphia, PA 19103
www.fadavis.com

Printed in the United States of America

Last digit indicates print number: 10 9 8 7 6 5 4 3 2

*Acquisitions Editor:*   Melanie Freely
*Developmental Editor:*   Catherine Harold
*Production Editor:*   Nwakaego Fletcher-Perry
*Cover Designer:*   Louis Forgione

As new scientific information becomes available through basic and clinical research, recommended treatments and drug therapies undergo changes. The author(s) and publisher have done everything possible to make this book accurate, up to date, and in accord with accepted standards at the time of publication. The author(s), editors, and publisher are not responsible for errors or omissions or for consequences from application of the book, and make no warranty, expressed or implied, in regard to the contents of the book. Any practice described in this book should be applied by the reader in accordance with professional standards of care used in regard to the unique circumstances that may apply in each situation. The reader is advised always to check product information (package inserts) for changes and new information regarding dose and contraindications before administering any drug. Caution is especially urged when using new or infrequently ordered drugs.

**Library of Congress Cataloging-in-Publication Data**

Schuster, Pamela McHugh, 1953-
    Concept mapping : a critical-thinking approach to care planning / Pamela McHugh Schuster.
        p. cm.
    Includes bibliographical references and index.
    ISBN 0-8036-0979-5 (pbk.)
    1. Nursing. 2. Critical thinking.    I. Title.
RT42 .S38 2002
362. 1'73'068—dc21

                                                                      2001047510

*This book is dedicated to nursing students*
*learning to organize patient-care planning and to provide effective nursing care,*
*and to the nursing students' clinical faculty.*

*Also to my husband,*
***Fred,***
*and my children,*
***Luke, Leeanna, Patty,*** *and* ***Isaac.***

## A NOTE ABOUT USAGE

To avoid both sexism and the constant repetition of "he or she," "his or her," and so forth, masculine and feminine pronouns are used alternately throughout the text.

# *Preface*

$\mathcal{D}$uring most of my 15 years as a clinical faculty member teaching foundations and medical-surgical nursing, I required my students to develop and submit weekly care plans using a five-column format common in nursing programs. I asked the students to complete as much of the care plan as possible before clinical, to come well prepared to the clinical preconference, and to submit to what some of them referred to as "Dr. Schuster's Grilling." The "grilling" consisted of me questioning them about their plans of care, which was highly frustrating for them and for me because most students have trouble summarizing patient data succinctly and developing comprehensive care plans from data.

For example, I once asked my students to assess a patient who had a hip replacement and to report the patient's priority problems in clinical preconference. One student reported that the patient's priority problem was a fever. I asked what caused the fever: Was it related to an infection in the surgical wound?, Was the patient developing atelectasis and pneumonia?, Or was the patient dehydrated and simply in need of fluids? The student could not tell. Consequently, she could not clearly determine what to do in response to the patient's fever. Another student stated that a priority problem was pain. I asked what caused the pain. Was it from the incision, from a backache caused by lying on the table for the procedure, or from a headache? Again, the student was not sure, so he had trouble determining an appropriate response to the problem.

One day out of frustration—the grilling was going very poorly—I asked my eight clinical students to write the main reason the patient needed health care in the center of a piece of paper and to arrange all of the patient's problems around that reason. I then told them to group all of the assessment data, the treatments, and the medications, as appropriate, under the problems they identified. The results were amazing. The students became organized in their thinking about problems and better understood the relationships in patient data. Once they better delineated specific problems, they were better able to discuss appropriate responses to those problems. They were thinking critically and coming up with wonderful ideas regarding patient-care planning and implementation of effective care. Performance in the clinical setting quickly improved, and the students were very pleased with themselves and with the care they provided.

Not long afterward, I described my students' success in care planning and clinical implementation to a colleague, who informed me that we were doing concept mapping. A review of the literature on concept mapping confirmed that my colleague was correct. I had discovered nothing new. Concept mapping is based on theories of learning and educational psychology. However, concept mapping is a new approach to teaching and learning about care planning in the health-care setting—an approach that nursing faculty and students agree is most exciting. Concept mapping is a diagrammatic teaching and learning strategy that allows students and faculty to visualize interrelationships between medical diagnoses, nursing diagnoses, assessment data, and treatments.

Before developing a concept map, the student must perform a comprehensive patient assessment. From the assessment data, the student develops a skeleton diagram of the patient's health problems (Step 1). The student then analyzes and categorizes specific patient assessment data (Step 2) and indicates relationships between nursing and medical diagnoses (Step 3). In Step 4, the student develops patient goals, outcomes, and nursing interventions for each nursing diagnosis. Step 5 is to evaluate the actual patient response to each nursing intervention and to summarize clinical impressions.

The result of Steps 1 through 4 is a holistic, comprehensive, and individualized plan of care that can be completed before patient care takes place. This visual map of problems and interventions is a personal pocket guide to patient care, and is the basis of nursing care discussions between students and faculty. Further, concept map care plans can be consulted throughout the clinical day, at the bedside, in the medication preparation area, and when preparing documentation. Concept map care planning evaluations have been excellent from both students and faculty.

This method of care planning is an alternative to the commonly used column format, which typically includes subjective and objective assessment data, nursing diagnoses, patient and family goals and outcomes, nursing interventions, rationales for the interventions, and evaluation of outcome objectives and goals. Nursing programs may vary slightly in what goes in each column, but until recently, the column format has been the typical way of teaching the nursing process and care planning in most programs. The problem is that these care plans are lengthy to write, time consuming, and commonly copied directly from a care planning book. They cannot realistically be completed before patient care, they focus on one problem at a time, and they fail to address the patient as a whole. Students report spending hours before and after clinical experiences writing care plans, and faculty report spending hours grading care plans. I'm convinced that concept map care planning offers a better way, and I wrote this book to help students learn to:

- Synthesize pertinent assessment data into comprehensive concept maps.
- Develop holistic and comprehensive care plans with nursing interventions that correspond to primary health problems and associated nursing diagnoses.
- Effectively implement nursing care using concept map care plans and thus improve clinical performance.

Concept maps help both faculty and students to clearly see patient needs, become quickly organized in thoughts and actions, and implement holistic care. They are practical, realistic, and time-saving. They reduce paperwork and improve clinical performance. Most importantly, they enhance critical-thinking skills and clinical reasoning because students can clearly and succinctly visualize priorities and identify relationships in patient data.

Recently, the critical-care faculty with whom I teach told me that they've started taping my students' concept map care plans to patients' bedside stands so they can use the diagrams as the focus of discussions between physicians, nurses, and students. Imagine a useful nursing care plan that both staff nurses and physicians favor, developed by student nurses! I wish you all much success in planning and implementing nursing care using this exciting new method of concept map care plans.

# Reviewers

**Emily Droste-Bielak**, RN, BSN, MS, PhD
Associate Professor
Grand Valley State University
Allendale, Michigan

**Linda Lea Kelly Brown**, RN, BSN, MA, MS, FNP-C
Professor
New Hampshire Community Technical College
Claremont, New Hampshire

**Sybil W. Damon**, RN, MS, DBA
VN Program Director
Summit Career College
Colton, California

**Dorcas C. Fitzgerald**, RN, MSN, DNSc
Professor and RN Track Coordinator
Department of Nursing
Youngstown State University
Youngstown, Ohio

**Joan Fleitas**
School of Nursing
Fairfield University
Fairfield, Connecticut

**Carole Heath**, RN, BSN, MSN, EdD, PHN
Professor
Sonoma State University
Rohnert Park, California

**Denise Landry**, RN, MSN, EdD, FNP
Professor, College of Nursing and Health Professions
Marshall University
Huntington, West Virginia

**Bonnie Raingruber**, RN, MS, PhD
Professor of Nursing
California State University
Sacramento, California

**Barbara Ann Ross**, RN, ASN, BSN, MSN, EdD
Assistant Professor and Web-developer
Indiana School of Nursing
Indianapolis, Indiana

**Peggy Wros**, RN, BSN, MSN, PhD
Associate Professor
Linfield College
Portland, Oregon

# Contents

# Chapter 1

## 'Twas the Night Before Clinical . . .

### OBJECTIVES

1. Define concept map care plans.

2. List the purposes of concept map care plans.

3. Identify the theoretical basis for clinical concept maps.

4. Relate critical-thinking processes to the nursing process and to concept map care plans.

5. Identify steps in the concept map care planning process.

6. Describe how concept map care planning corresponds to the nursing process.

7. Identify how concept map care plans are used during patient care.

8. Describe the purpose of standards of care as related to care planning.

9. List health-care providers and agencies responsible for developing and enforcing standards of care.

10. Describe the purpose of managed care.

'Twas the night before clinical and all through the house, not a creature was stirring . . . except for you! There you are with books piled high around you trying to get ready to give safe and competent nursing care to the patients you have been assigned in the morning. It is late, and you are tired. What if there were a way for all the information you have gathered on your patients to just "come together," make perfect sense, and form a simple, complete care plan? If you have ever found yourself in this situation, this book is for you. It was written to help you quickly and efficiently organize and analyze patient data and develop a working care plan. The plans you develop will be practical and realistic; they will be implemented and evaluated during the clinical day. And best of all, there is very little writing to do! No more tedious writing of nursing care plans!

The purpose of this chapter is to describe the theoretical basis for concept map care plans and to provide an overview of what concept map care plans are, how they are developed, and how they are used during patient care. In addition, the chapter introduces general standards for guiding and evaluating patient care within managed care systems. Managed care principles are used in almost all health-care delivery systems. The purpose of managed care is to decrease costs while maintaining the quality of health-care services. The implications of managed care regarding care planning are far-reaching, and they guide the development of nursing care plans. Later chapters will lead you step by step through each aspect of developing and using concept map care plans.

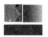 ## WHAT ARE CONCEPT MAP CARE PLANS?

The concept map care plan is an innovative approach to planning and organizing nursing care. In essence, a concept map care plan is a diagram of patient problems and interventions. Your ideas about patient problems and treatments are the "concepts" that will be diagrammed. In this book, the term *concept* means idea. You will diagram your ideas about the patient's problems and their treatments. Developing clinical concept map care plans will enhance your critical thinking skills and clinical reasoning because you will clearly and succinctly visualize priorities and identify relationships in clinical patient data. Concept map care plans are used to organize patient data, analyze relationships in the data, establish priorities, build on previous knowledge, identify what you do not understand, and enable you to take a holistic view of the patient's situation.

 ## THE THEORETICAL BASIS OF CONCEPT MAP CARE PLANNING

Concept map care plans have roots in the fields of education and psychology.[1,2] Concept maps have also been called cognitive maps, mind maps, and meta-cognitive tools for teaching/learning.[3,4] Nursing educators have recognized the usefulness of this teaching/learning strategy in summarizing and visualizing important concepts, and there is a growing body of knowledge on this topic.[5-9]

From the field of education, Novak and Gowin[10] developed the theory of meaningful learning and have written about "learning how to learn." They have theoretically defined concept maps as "schematic devices for representing a set of concept meanings embedded in a framework of propositions." They further explain concept maps as hierarchical graphical organizers that serve to demonstrate the understanding of relationships among concepts. This theoretical definition and explanation is highly abstract. Simply stated, concept maps are diagrams of important ideas that are linked together. The important ideas you need to link are patient problems and treatments for those problems.

The educational psychologist Ausubel[11] has also contributed to the theoretical basis of concept mapping through the development of assimilation theory. Concept maps help those who write them to assimilate knowledge. The premise of this theory is that new knowledge is built on preexisting knowledge structures, and new concepts are integrated by identifying relationships with those concepts already understood. Simply stated, we build and integrate new knowledge into what we already know. Through diagramming in a concept map, you build the structure of what is known about the relationships in a concept. Thus, concept maps help to identify and integrate what you already know. In addition, concept maps can help reveal what you do not understand. This means that although you have ideas about patient problems or treatments, you may not be sure of how those problems and treatments should be integrated into a comprehensive plan. Once you recognize what you do not understand and can formulate questions, you can seek out information. Concept maps will help identify what you know about patient care and what you need to learn to provide quality care.

Concept mapping requires critical thinking. A widely accepted view of critical thinking by many nurse educators was developed by the

American Philosophical Association: "Critical thinking is the process of purposeful, self-regulatory judgment. This process gives reasoned consideration to evidence, contexts, conceptualization, methods, and criteria."[12] In developing a clinical concept map care plan, critical thinking is used to analyze relationships in clinical data. Thus, critical thinking used in developing concept map care plans builds clinical reasoning skills. Critical thinking and clinical reasoning are used to formulate clinical judgments and decisions about nursing care.

Although concept maps have been used in a number of different ways in various disciplines including nursing, the focus of this book is on developing concept maps for the purposes of clinical nursing care planning. The important ideas that must be linked together during clinical care planning are the medical and nursing diagnoses, along with all pertinent clinical data. Concept map care planning can be used to promote critical thinking and clinical reasoning about patient problems and treatment of problems. Through concept mapping of diagnoses and clinical data, you can evaluate what you know about the care of a patient and what further information you need to provide safe and effective nursing care. The visual map of relationships among diagnoses allows you and your clinical faculty to exchange views on why relationships exist among diagnoses. It also allows you to recognize missing diagnoses and linkages, thus suggesting a need for further learning.

## OVERVIEW OF STEPS IN CONCEPT MAP CARE PLANNING

The nursing process is foundational to developing and using the concept map care plan or any other type of nursing care plan. The nursing process involves assessing, diagnosing, planning, implementing, and evaluating nursing care. These steps of the nursing process are related to the development of concept map care plans and the use of care plans during patient care in clinical settings. Subsequent chapters will give the details of concept map care planning with learning activities, but it is important for you to have an initial overview.

## ■ Preparation for Concept Mapping

Before developing a concept map, the first thing you must do is gather clinical data. This step corresponds to the assessment phase of the nursing process. You must review patient records to determine current health problems, medical histories, physical assessment data, medications, and treatments. This assessment must be complete and accurate because it forms the basis for the concept map. Some of you may have the opportunity to briefly meet patients the night before you care for them. In just five minutes of interacting with a patient—even by simply introducing yourself and watching the patient's response—you can gain a wealth of information about the patient's mood, level of comfort, and ability to communicate. Chapter 2 will focus on how to gather this clinical data in preparation for developing a concept map.

## ■ Step 1: Develop a Basic Skeleton Diagram

Based on the clinical data you collect, you begin a concept map care plan by developing a basic skeleton diagram of the reasons your patient needs health care. The initial diagram is composed of clinical impressions you make after reviewing all of the data. Write the patient's reason for seeking care (usually a medical diagnosis) in the middle of a blank sheet of paper. Then, around this central diagnosis, arrange general problems (nursing diagnoses) that represent patient responses to the patient's specific reason for seeking health care as shown in Figure 1–1. The general problem statements will eventually be written as nursing diagnoses as shown in Figure 1–1.[13]

The American Nurses Association (ANA) Social Policy Statement[14] indicates that the focus of nursing practice is on human responses to health states. The map reflects the ANA practice policy statement because the human responses are located around the health state of the patient. Nursing care will be focused on the human responses.

The central figure of the map is whatever reason the patient is seeking health care—the reason for the hospitalization, extended care, or visit to the outpatient center. In Figure 1–1, the health problem for which a patient seeks care,

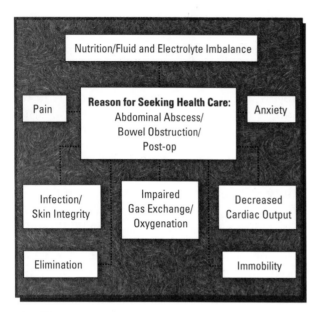

**■ *Figure* 1–1**

**Nursing and medical diagnoses.**

the medical diagnosis, is centrally located on the map. However, the central figure may not always contain a medical diagnosis: Sometimes the focus of a visit may be on high-level wellness, when the patient will be seen for a screening examination, and the aim is to maintain wellness and prevent problems.

The map is primarily composed of nursing diagnoses resulting from the health state, flowing outward from the central figure like spokes on a wheel. The map focuses strictly on real nursing care problems based on collected data. It does not focus on potential problems. At this stage of care planning, it is most important to recognize major problem areas. You do not have to state the nursing diagnosis yet. Write down your general impressions of the patient after your initial review of data.

Labeling the correct diagnosis is difficult for many students. However, at this point, it is more important to recognize major problem areas than to worry about the correct nursing diagnostic label. If you recognize that the patient has a major problem breathing, write it down. You are trying to get the big picture here. Later, you can look up the correct nursing diagnostic label and decide if the diagnosis should be **Impaired Gas Ex-**change, **Ineffective Airway Clearance,** or **Ineffective Breathing Patterns.** Initially, just write, in whatever words come to mind, what you think are the patient's problems. Recognizing that something is wrong with the patient is more important than applying the correct label. Step 1 on formulating basic diagrams of problems will be expanded on in Chapter 3.

## ■ Step 2: Analyze and Categorize Data

In this step, you must analyze and categorize data gathered from the patient's medical records and your brief encounter with the patient. By categorizing the data, you provide evidence to support the medical and nursing diagnoses. You must identify and group the most important assessment data related to the patient's reason for seeking health care. You must also identify and group clinical assessment data, treatments, medications, and medical history data related to the nursing diagnoses, as shown in Figure 1–2.[15]

In this example of a concept map, you see the nursing diagnoses flowing outward from the patient's reason for seeking health care. Listed within each nursing diagnosis is the clinical evidence of problems that led the creator of the map to conclude that the diagnosis was important for that patient at that time.

Thus, when making a concept map care plan, you must write important clinical assessment data, treatments, medications, and medical history data related to each nursing diagnosis. This involves sifting through and sorting out the often-voluminous amount of data that you collected on your patient. The sicker the patient, the more complex the analysis. You need to list assessment data regarding physical and emotional indicators of problems or symptoms under the appropriate diagnoses. For example, physical indicators of problems from the data include labored respirations at a rate of 22, fatigue, and decreased breath sounds. These are listed under the nursing diagnosis **Impaired Gas Exchange**. Emotional indicators of problems include the patient crying and verbalizing that he is nervous and saying that he knows he is going to die. These are listed under the nursing diagnosis **Anxiety**.

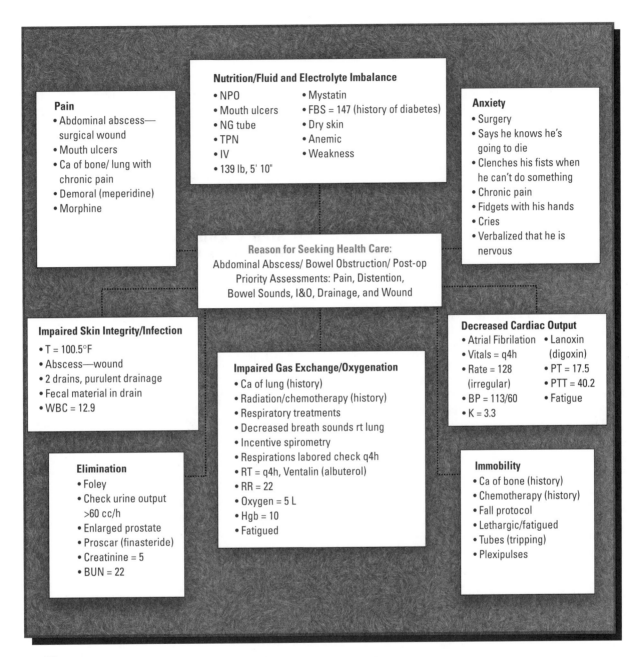

**Pain**
- Abdominal abscess—surgical wound
- Mouth ulcers
- Ca of bone/ lung with chronic pain
- Demoral (meperidine)
- Morphine

**Nutrition/Fluid and Electrolyte Imbalance**
- NPO
- Mouth ulcers
- NG tube
- TPN
- IV
- 139 lb, 5' 10"
- Mystatin
- FBS = 147 (history of diabetes)
- Dry skin
- Anemic
- Weakness

**Anxiety**
- Surgery
- Says he knows he's going to die
- Clenches his fists when he can't do something
- Chronic pain
- Fidgets with his hands
- Cries
- Verbalized that he is nervous

**Reason for Seeking Health Care:**
Abdominal Abscess/ Bowel Obstruction/ Post-op
Priority Assessments: Pain, Distention,
Bowel Sounds, I&O, Drainage, and Wound

**Impaired Skin Integrity/Infection**
- T = 100.5°F
- Abscess—wound
- 2 drains, purulent drainage
- Fecal material in drain
- WBC = 12.9

**Impaired Gas Exchange/Oxygenation**
- Ca of lung (history)
- Radiation/chemotherapy (history)
- Respiratory treatments
- Decreased breath sounds rt lung
- Incentive spirometry
- Respirations labored check q4h
- RT = q4h, Ventalin (albuterol)
- RR = 22
- Oxygen = 5 L
- Hgb = 10
- Fatigued

**Decreased Cardiac Output**
- Atrial Fibrilation
- Vitals = q4h
- Rate = 128 (irregular)
- BP = 113/60
- K = 3.3
- Lanoxin (digoxin)
- PT = 17.5
- PTT = 40.2
- Fatigue

**Elimination**
- Foley
- Check urine output >60 cc/h
- Enlarged prostate
- Proscar (finasteride)
- Creatinine = 5
- BUN = 22

**Immobility**
- Ca of bone (history)
- Chemotherapy (history)
- Fall protocol
- Lethargic/fatigued
- Tubes (tripping)
- Plexipulses

■ *Figure* **1–2**

**Data to support diagnoses. Ca = cancer; BP = blood pressure; BUN = blood urea nitrogen; FBS = fasting blood sugar; Hgb = hemoglobin; I&O = intake and output; IV = intravenous; K = potassium; NG = nasogastric; NPO = nothing by mouth; PT = prothrombin time; PTT = partial thromboplastin time; RR = respiratory rate; RT = respiratory therapy; T = temperature; TPN = total parenteral nutrition; WBCs = white blood cells.**

You must also list current information on diagnostic test data, treatments, and medications under the appropriate nursing diagnoses. You may need to look up the diagnostic tests, treatments, and medications if you are not familiar with them. You must think critically to place diagnostic test data, treatments, and medications under the appropriate category. For example, diagnostic tests include blood studies of white blood cells, hemoglobin, and potassium. In this case, the white blood cells are listed with **Infection**, the hemoglobin with **Oxygenation**, and the potassium with **Decreased Cardiac Output**. Oxygen and respiratory treatments are categorized with **Impaired Gas Exchange**. The medication Demerol (meperidine) is categorized with **Pain**, while Ventolin (albuterol) is categorized with **Impaired Gas Exchange**, and Lanoxin (digoxin) with **Decreased Cardiac Output**.

You must also list medical history information under the nursing diagnoses. In this example, the patient has a history of bone and lung cancer, atrial fibrillation, and an enlarged prostate. The bone and lung cancer history is listed under the nursing diagnoses of **Pain**, **Gas Exchange**, and **Immobility**; atrial fibrillation is under **Decreased Cardiac Output**, and the enlarged prostate is listed under **Elimination**.

When beginning to use concept maps with medical and nursing diagnoses that are new to you, you may not always know where to categorize an abnormal symptom, laboratory value, treatment, drug, or history information. If you do not know where the data should go but you think it is important, list it off to the side of the map and ask for clarification from your clinical faculty. At least you recognized it was important; you do not yet have the experience to see where the data fits in the overall clinical picture of patient care.

Sometimes you may think that symptoms apply to more than one nursing diagnosis, and they often do. You may recognize that the patient is lethargic and fatigued, but that observation could go under **Decreased Cardiac Output**, **Immobility**, **Nutrition**, or **Decreased Gas Exchange**. It makes sense to place this symptom in more than one area. Therefore, you can repeat a symptom in different categories if it is relevant to more than one category.

Finally, determine the priority assessments that still need to be performed regarding the primary reason for seeking care (the primary medical diagnosis); write them in the box at the center of the map as shown in Figure 1–2. These priority assessments must be done on first contact with the patient and carefully monitored throughout the clinical day. Focus on the key areas of physical assessment that must be performed to ensure safe patient care. This step in the concept map care planning process appears in detail in Chapter 3.

## ■ Step 3: Analyze Nursing Diagnoses Relationships

Next, you need to analyze relationships among the nursing diagnoses. Draw lines between nursing diagnoses to indicate relationships as shown in Figure 1–3.[17] In this example, pain is related to **Anxiety**, **Immobility**, **Infection**, and **Nutrition**. Be prepared to verbally explain to your clinical faculty why you have made these links if it is not obvious. For example, why pain and nutrition? In this case, the explanation is that the patient has mouth ulcers and an uncomfortable nasogastric tube, contributing to pain. You will soon recognize that all the problems the patient is having are interrelated. You and your clinical faculty can see the "whole picture" of what is happening with the patient by looking at the map. Thus, concept mapping is a holistic approach to patient care. Step 3 focuses on the relationships between diagnoses and the labeling of nursing diagnoses according to the North American Nursing Diagnosis Association classification system (see Appendix C). These issues will be expanded upon in Chapter 3. Also, you will number each nursing diagnosis on the map.

## ■ Step 4: Identifying Goals, Outcomes, and Interventions

Then, on a separate sheet of paper, you will write patient goals and outcomes and then list nursing interventions to attain the outcomes for each of the numbered diagnoses on your map. This step, which corresponds to the planning phase of the nursing process, is shown in the first column of Box 1–1.[18]

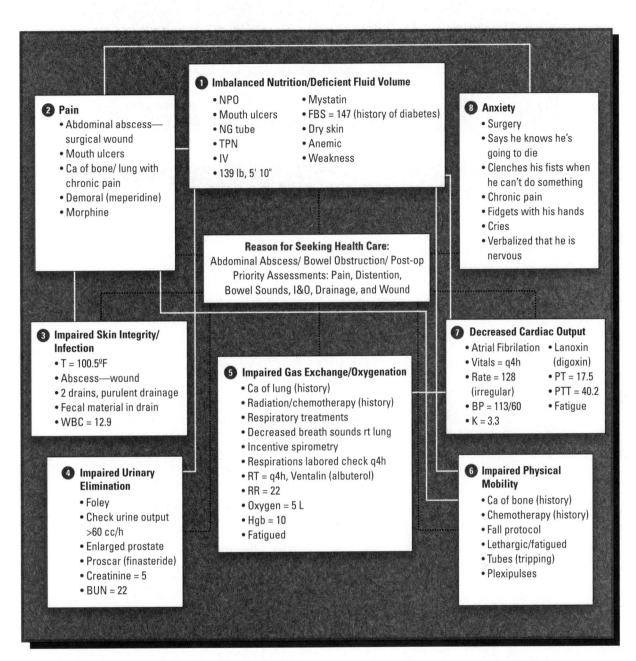

**1 Imbalanced Nutrition/Deficient Fluid Volume**
- NPO
- Mouth ulcers
- NG tube
- TPN
- IV
- 139 lb, 5' 10"
- Mystatin
- FBS = 147 (history of diabetes)
- Dry skin
- Anemic
- Weakness

**2 Pain**
- Abdominal abscess—surgical wound
- Mouth ulcers
- Ca of bone/ lung with chronic pain
- Demoral (meperidine)
- Morphine

**8 Anxiety**
- Surgery
- Says he knows he's going to die
- Clenches his fists when he can't do something
- Chronic pain
- Fidgets with his hands
- Cries
- Verbalized that he is nervous

**Reason for Seeking Health Care:**
Abdominal Abscess/ Bowel Obstruction/ Post-op
Priority Assessments: Pain, Distention,
Bowel Sounds, I&O, Drainage, and Wound

**3 Impaired Skin Integrity/ Infection**
- T = 100.5ºF
- Abscess—wound
- 2 drains, purulent drainage
- Fecal material in drain
- WBC = 12.9

**5 Impaired Gas Exchange/Oxygenation**
- Ca of lung (history)
- Radiation/chemotherapy (history)
- Respiratory treatments
- Decreased breath sounds rt lung
- Incentive spirometry
- Respirations labored check q4h
- RT = q4h, Ventalin (albuterol)
- RR = 22
- Oxygen = 5 L
- Hgb = 10
- Fatigued

**7 Decreased Cardiac Output**
- Atrial Fibrillation
- Vitals = q4h
- Rate = 128 (irregular)
- BP = 113/60
- K = 3.3
- Lanoxin (digoxin)
- PT = 17.5
- PTT = 40.2
- Fatigue

**4 Impaired Urinary Elimination**
- Foley
- Check urine output >60 cc/h
- Enlarged prostate
- Proscar (finasteride)
- Creatinine = 5
- BUN = 22

**6 Impaired Physical Mobility**
- Ca of bone (history)
- Chemotherapy (history)
- Fall protocol
- Lethargic/fatigued
- Tubes (tripping)
- Plexipulses

■ *Figure* 1–3

Relationships between diagnoses. Ca = cancer; BP = blood pressure; BUN = blood urea nitrogen; FBS = fasting blood sugar; Hgb = hemoglobin; I&O = intake and output; IV = intravenous; K = potassium; NG = nasogastric; NPO = nothing by mouth; PT = prothrombin time; PTT = partial thromboplastin time; RR = respiratory rate; RT = respiratory therapy; T = temperature; TPN = total parenteral nutrition; WBCs = white blood cells

## Box 1-1    PHYSICAL AND PSYCHOSOCIAL RESPONSES

**Problem No. 1:**  Imbalanced Nutrition, Imbalanced Fluid Volume
**Goal:**  Improve nutrition
**Outcome:**  Patient's NG, TPN, and JP drains will remain patent, and patient's intake of fluids and electrolytes will balance outputs.

| STEP 4 | STEP 5 |
|---|---|
| **Nursing Nutrition/Fluid Interventions** | **Patient Responses (Evaluation)** |
| 1. Assess new lab values | 1. No new lab values except as shown below |
| 2. Assess I&O | 2. Intake 600/ Output 650 |
| 3. NPO | 3. NPO except ice and medications |
| 4. Mouth care with nystatin mouth wash | 4. Liked the taste, said it helped a lot |
| 5. Ice chips | 5. Sucked on for sore throat |
| 6. Monitor NG tube, check drainage | 6. Nurse checked (skill not yet learned) |
| 7. Monitor TPN | 7. Nurse checked (skill not yet learned) |
| 8. Assess FBS | 8. 109 at 6 A.M. |
| 9. Assess abdominal pain | 9. Grimacing, moaning, "5" |
| 10. Morphine for pain | 10. Gave MS at 8:40; "2" at 9:15 |
| 11. Bowel sounds | 11. Hypoactive |
| 12. Distention | 12. None, soft (has NG tube) |
| 13. Skin turgor | 13. Poor, dry. Lubricated with bath |
| 14. Drainage, JP | 14. Purulent yellow, foul-smelling A− and purulent green B− |

*Impressions: Nutritional status in balance with intake equal to output, electrolytes stable, tubes remain patent, bowels remain hypoactive.*

**Problem No. 2:**  Pain
**Goal:**  Control pain
**Outcome:**  Patient's pain remains below 3 on a 10-point scale.

| STEP 4 | STEP 5 |
|---|---|
| **Nursing Pain Interventions** | **Patient Responses (Evaluation)** |
| 1. Assess pain with scale and medicate with | 1. As above |
| 2. Demerol (meperidine) and morphine | 2. "   " |
| 3. Positioning | 3. Positioned with pillow in bed |
| 4. Check noise, lighting | 4. Decreased light and fell asleep |
| 5. Guided Imagery | 5. Visualized a beach |
| 6. Backrub | 6. Stated it hurt to be touched |

*Impressions: Patient needs narcotics to control pain and likes the nondrug measures of positioning, noise and light control, and guided imagery.*

**Box 1–1** | *PHYSICAL AND PSYCHOSOCIAL RESPONSES (CONTINUED)*

**Problem No. 3:** Infection, Impaired Skin Integrity
**Goal:** Prevent further infection
**Outcome:** The patient's infection will not get any worse and temperature will remain WNL.

| STEP 4 | STEP 5 |
| --- | --- |
| **Nursing Infection Control Interventions** | **Patient Responses (Evaluation)** |
| 1. Monitor temperature | 1. 96.2°F at 8 A.M., 97.9°F at 12 P.M. |
| 2. Assess WBC | 2. No new values |
| 3. Bed bath | 3. Cooperated but had pain as above |
| 4. Check skin integrity | 4. No signs of additional breakdown |
| 5. Clean Foley | 5. Patent, skin pink, and intact |
| 6. Oral care | 6. Mouth sores; used nystatin |
| 7. Assess wounds, drains | 7. Intact, no redness or edema—drains above |

*Impressions: Drainage from drains looks purulent, although incision intact without s/s of infection, temperature WNL*

**Problem No. 4:** Impaired Urinary Elimination
**Goal:** Maintain elimination
**Outcome:** The urine output will be >60 cc/h.

| STEP 4 | STEP 5 |
| --- | --- |
| **Nursing Elimination Interventions** | **Patient Responses (Evaluation)** |
| 1. Call physician if urine output <60 cc/h | 1. >60 cc/h |
| 2. Check Foley patency | 2. Patent, draining |
| 3. Check color, amount, smell | 3. Clear, yellow, no smell |
| 4. Clean Foley | 4. As above |
| 5. Bedpan for BMs | 5. None |
| 6. I&O | 6. As above |
| 7. Monitor BUN, creatinine | 7. No new labs drawn |

*Impressions: Patient's elimination maintained above 60 cc/h.*

**Problem No. 5:** Impaired Gas Exchange
**Goal:** Maintain oxygenation
**Outcome:** Patient cooperates with RT, uses oxygen, and breathing remains nonlabored.

| STEP 4 | STEP 5 |
| --- | --- |
| **Nursing Oxygenation Interventions** | **Patient Responses** |
| 1. Monitor breath sounds | 1. Rales throughout especially rt base |
| 2. Check VS, especially respirations | 2. 8 A.M. 156/80; 96.2°F; 112; 20 |
|  | 12 P.M. 126/58; 97.4°F; 88; 20 |
| 3. Do CDB with respiratory therapist (RT) | 3. RT did CDB after treatments |
| 4. Oxygen intact | 4. Tolerated well |
|  | On at 5 L |
| 5. Fatigue | 5. See immobility |
| 6. Monitor Hgb | 6. No new labs |

*Impressions: Breathing nonlabored but remains congested, cooperative with treatments, elevations in BP and pulse probably due to pain as above.*

*(Continued)*

| **Box 1–1** | *PHYSICAL AND PSYCHOSOCIAL RESPONSES (CONTINUED)* |
|---|---|

**Problem No. 6:**  Impaired Physical Mobility
　　　**Goal:**  Maintain movements
　**Outcome:**  Patient performs ROM, gets up to chair, remains free from injury.

| STEP 4 | STEP 5 |
|---|---|
| **Nursing Mobility Interventions** | **Patient Responses (Evaluation)** |
| 1. Monitor fatigue | 1. Weak and tired |
| 2. Safe environment (fall protocol) | 2. Personal items in reach |
| 3. Side rails, bed low, call bell in reach | 3. At all times |
| 4. Compression devices on in bed | 4. On for 2 h |
| 5. Do ROM | 5. Did ROM with bath |
| 6. Get up in chair at bedside | 6. Up for 1 h and became fatigued |

*Impressions: Got up for an hour but is weak and tired. Performed ROM. High potential for a fall due to weakness and fatigue.*

**Problem No. 7:**  Decreased Cardiac Output
　　　**Goal:**  Maintain cardiac output
　**Outcome:**  Pulse and BP remain stable and electrolytes WNL.

| STEP 4 | STEP 5 |
|---|---|
| **Nursing Cardiac Output Interventions** | **Patient Responses (Evaluation)** |
| 1. Check VS q4h, especially BP and P | 1. As above |
| 2. Apical check with digoxin (Lanoxin) | 2. 112 at 10 A.M. |
| 3. Check K | 3. K = 3.8 |
| 4. Listen for arrythmias | 4. None noted |

*Impressions: BP and P elevations probably due to pain; CV system appears stable.*

**Problem No. 8:**  Anxiety
　　　**Goal:**  Decrease anxiety
　**Outcome:**  Patient verbalizes concerns.

| STEP 4 | STEP 5 |
|---|---|
| **Nursing Anxiety Interventions** | **Patient Responses (Evaluation)** |
| 1. Guided imagery | 1. States that it is relaxing |
| 2. Therapeutic communication, especially empathy, distraction, active listening | 2. Verbalized concerns |
| 3. Comfort touch | 3. Held my hand when talking |
| 4. Teach slow deep-breathing | 4. Appeared more relaxed, less grimacing |

*Impressions: Patient responded to anxiety interventions by verbalizing concerns.*

Key: BUN = blood urea nitrogen; BM = bowel movement; CDB = cough and deep breathing; FBS = fasting blood sugar; JP = juvenile periodontitis; NG = nasogastric; P = pulse; ROM = range of motion; TPN = total parenteral nutrition; VS = vital signs; WBCs = white blood cells; WNL = within normal limits.

You must list the nursing care you intend to provide for the patient during the time that you are scheduled to be interacting with the patient. You will carry the map and list of interventions in your pocket as you work with the patient, and you will either check off interventions as you complete them or make revisions in the diagram and interventions as you interact with the patient. The map and interventions are used during the intervention phase of the nursing process.

The nursing interventions include key areas of assessment and monitoring as well as procedures or other therapeutic interventions such as patient teaching or therapeutic communication. To decrease paperwork, the goals and rationales for interventions are not written down. Come prepared to verbally explain the goals and rationales for your identified nursing actions if asked by your clinical faculty. It is of course a professional responsibility to know why you are doing each action, even though you are not writing it down.

Be prepared to review nursing interventions during clinical pre-conferencing. Nursing interventions include what you are supposed to be carefully monitoring. In addition, nursing interventions should include a list of all appropriate treatments and medications. Patient teaching should be listed under nursing interventions as appropriate for each problem. For example, patient teaching may involve slow, deep breathing and guided imagery under the nursing diagnosis **Anxiety**.

If you have not yet learned how to perform a treatment but you know the treatment needs to be done, list it in the nursing intervention column, and also note that the nurse assigned to oversee the patient's care will be doing the treatment. For example, under nutrition, you may write that the patient needs total parenteral nutrition and care of the nasogastric tube, but that these services will be done by the staff nurse since you have not yet learned how to provide them. By writing down the treatments in the appropriate column, you demonstrate that you have recognized these nutrition-related treatments and that they are important aspects of the total care needed by the patient. Be prepared to discuss the basic purpose of the interventions, even those you do not perform yourself. Step 4

on outcomes and nursing interventions will be expanded on in Chapter 4.

 ## Step 5: Evaluate Patient's Responses

This step is the written evaluation of the patient's physical and psychosocial responses. It is shown in the second column of Box 1–1.[19] As you perform a nursing activity, write down patient's responses. For example, you said that you would monitor the patient's temperature in Step 4 under the nursing diagnosis **Infection**. In Step 5, you record those temperatures across from the intervention. Step 5 also involves writing your clinical impressions and inferences regarding the patient's progress toward expected outcomes and the effectiveness of your interventions to bring these outcomes about. This is a summary statement written for each nursing diagnosis, found at the end of each intervention and response list. Step 5 on evaluation of outcomes will be expanded on in Chapters 5 and 6.

## DURING CLINICAL CARE: KEEP IT IN YOUR POCKET

Throughout the clinical day, you and your clinical faculty will have an ongoing discussion regarding changes in patient assessment data, effectiveness of interventions, and patient responses to those interventions. Keep the map and list of interventions in your pocket; this way, everything that must be done and evaluated is listed succinctly and kept within easy reach. As the plan is revised throughout the day, take notes on the map, add or delete nursing interventions, and write patient responses as you go along. As your clinical faculty makes rounds and checks in on you and your patients, the faculty can also refer to the maps and intervention lists you have developed as the basis for guiding your patient care.

 ## DOCUMENTATION

The maps, interventions, and patient responses will become the basis of your documentation.

You will be using the revised plans and outcome evaluations as guides to make sure you have adequately documented patient problems, interventions, and the evaluation of patient responses. Documentation involves correctly identifying patient assessment data to record about a problem, determining what to record about the interventions to correct the problem, and describing the patient's responses to the interventions. Assessment, interventions, and responses are all present in the concept map care plan. Concept map care plans as the basis of documentation will be described in more detail in Chapter 7.

 **MEDICATION ADMINISTRATION**

Your concept map care plan will also be useful as you prepare to administer medications. By organizing the drugs to be administered under the correct problem, you demonstrate your knowledge of the relationship of the drug to the problem. You can also see the interactive effects of the drug related to the total clinical picture. For example, as you discuss Lanoxin (digitalis) administration under **Decreased Cardiac Output,** you and your clinical faculty can also see that the patient's potassium level was low. What is the relationship between low levels of potassium and Lanoxin administration? The answer is an increased risk of a toxic reaction by the patient to digitalis. Be prepared for your clinical faculty to ask you for the current value of potassium from the morning blood draw. Low potassium levels have to be corrected; in the meantime, you can be assessing the patient carefully for adverse reactions to the drug. You can more easily integrate medications with laboratory values and pathology if the information is all neatly categorized under decreased cardiac output.

In addition, you should also write down scheduled times of medication administration next to the drugs. You may also highlight drugs on the map. Writing down administration times and highlighting drugs helps to organize, and remind you of the importance of, the medication administration times. It also decreases the chance of medication errors.

 **NURSING STANDARDS OF CARE**

Concept map care plans are individualized plans of care built on critical analysis of patient assessment data, identification of medical and nursing diagnoses, determination of nursing actions to be implemented, and evaluation of patient responses. Development, implementation, and evaluation of safe and effective nursing care are contingent upon nurses knowing and following accepted standards of care. As you plan care for a patient, a primary question you must address is this: What are the standards of care pertinent to my patient and specific to the applicable medical and nursing diagnoses? Nursing students often wonder: "Have I included everything necessary in this care plan?" "Am I doing everything I should be doing?" "Am I missing something?" Following standards of care ensures that you are doing everything possible to provide appropriate care to the patient. These standards may stem from several organizing agencies or principles.

### Standards of the American Nurses Association

By law, nurses must follow guidelines for the safe and effective practice of nursing. These legal guidelines are called *standards of care.* The ANA has developed general standards of nursing practice, shown in Box 1–2.[20] Concept map care plans are in compliance with these general standards of care.

### Standards of the Joint Commission on Accreditation of Healthcare Organizations

In addition, there are also very specific standards to be followed when caring for patients with specific problems. The Joint Commission on Accreditation of Healthcare Organizations (JCAHO) requires that all accredited agencies have written policies and procedures for nursing care. You must follow these specific policies and procedures for any nursing care you administer. Representatives of JCAHO travel the country and review these policies and procedures. If they are not current, JCAHO requires that they be up-

> ### Box 1–2    AMERICAN NURSES ASSOCIATION STANDARDS OF CLINICAL NURSING PRACTICE
>
> 1. The collection of data about the health status of the patient is systematic and continuous. The data are accessible, communicated and recorded.
>
> 2. Nursing diagnoses are derived from health status data, validated and documented.
>
> 3. The nurse identifies expected outcomes derived from the nursing diagnoses.
>
> 4. The nurse develops a plan of nursing care including priorities and the prescribed nursing approaches or measures to achieve the outcomes derived from the nursing diagnoses. Nursing interventions provide for patient participation in health promotion, maintenance, and restoration.
>
> 5. The nurse implements and documents interventions consistent with the plan of care.
>
> 6. The patient and the nurse determine the patient's progress or lack of progress toward outcome achievement and documents accordingly. The patient's progress or lack of progress toward goal achievement directs reassessment, reordering of priorities, new goal setting and revision of the plan of nursing care.
>
> SOURCE: Standards of Clinical Nursing Practice, ed 2. American Nurses Publishing, American Nurses Foundation/American Nurses Association, Washington, D.C., 1998, with permission.

dated if the agency desires to maintain its certification.

Fortunately for you as a student, fundamentals and medical-surgical textbooks provide general descriptions of procedures similar to what is required by your clinical agency. Your clinical faculty will inform you of any specific requirements of the clinical agency in which you are placed, either by explaining those requirements verbally or referring you to the agency's procedure manual.

### ▥ Standardized Nursing Care Plans

Many organizations have developed standardized nursing care plans for specific medical diagnoses. These standardized nursing care plans are based on typical nursing diagnoses of patients with particular medical problems. Many facilities have general nursing care plans for nursing care of patients that are commonly seen at the site. For example, an orthopedic unit probably has a standardized care plan for the patient with a fractured hip, and the urology unit probably has a standardized care plan for the patient undergoing a transurethral resection of the prostate gland. In addition, hundreds of standardized care plans have been written and published, and many have been computerized for easy accessibility.

Therefore, while you are gathering data from a patient's records to prepare your concept map care plan, you also need to find out whether the agency has any standardized care plans available for you to use. If these plans are not available on the unit to which you are assigned, you can use published standardized care plan books to make sure you have not missed any important aspects of care.

### ▥ Patient Education Standards

All patients have the right to know what is wrong with them and how to manage their own care. That makes patient education a key role for nurses. Most agencies have patient education materials available that are specific to various types of problems. You also need to collect these materials when you collect information from patient records. As with standardized care plans, there are also published standardized teaching materials, such as booklets and movies, that may be available for you and the patient as references. Teaching materials are usually geared toward a fifth-grade reading level. Materials given to patients must be carefully screened for content that is appropriate for the patient's individual needs and ability to comprehend the materials. Detailed information about integrating teaching materials with concept map care plans appears in later chapters.

## ■ Insurance Agency and Government Care Standards

The high cost of health care has led to a concerted effort by the government (which pays for Medicare and Medicaid) and health-care insurance companies to control costs. At the same time that costs are being controlled, the quality of health care is supposed to be ensured through careful management by health-care providers. The government and insurance companies have developed specific criteria for which services will and will not be reimbursed, depending on diagnoses. All medications, treatments, surgeries, and rehabilitation programs (literally everything done by health-care providers) has to be provided and documented according to government and insurance company criteria for care, or the bills will not be paid. When bills are not paid by the government or insurance companies, health-care providers may never receive payment for services provided. In some cases, patients may be left with the bill. In that case, patients may decide to go without needed health-care services because they cannot afford them.

Insurance companies and the government pay predetermined amounts of money to agencies or physicians providing care to patients. For example, if a patient had knee replacement surgery, the providers will receive a fixed amount of money for that service. Case managers, typically advanced practice nurses, are hired by insurance companies and health-care agencies to evaluate the types of care given to inpatients and outpatients, to monitor patient progress, and coordinate the care of patients to guide their recovery while minimizing costs. These case managers are also known as resource managers, because they coordinate all services available to the patient. They must be aware of all resources available so they can make the appropriate linkages between patients and the appropriate services.

Teams of health-care providers including physicians, nurses, pharmacists, dietitians, physical therapists, and social workers have developed standards that guide the treatment of patients. Instead of separate plans of care from the physician, dietitian, and others, the trend is for health-care providers to collaborate and develop one unified plan of care. This multidisciplinary plan is commonly called a *clinical pathway* or a *critical pathway*. There is careful sequencing of clinical interventions over a specific period of time that all involved in the care of the patient agree to follow. Clinical pathways outline assessments, treatments, procedures, diet, activities, patient education, and discharge planning activities. Although clinical pathways are becoming a popular method of collaborative care planning, they are unfortunately not available for every diagnosis. Clinical pathways also vary slightly among clinical agencies.

As you prepare for a clinical care assignment, it is important that you know about the clinical pathway your patient is supposed to be following based on the patient's health condition. Since nurses often spend more time with patients than other health-care providers, nurses' clinical roles include communicating between caregivers to make sure that the patient is making steady progress in the expected direction toward health goals enumerated on the clinical pathway. The nursing care plan and assessment is focused on identifying complications and quickly intervening to get the patient back on the clinical pathway to resume rapid progress toward health goals.

Currently, a battle is raging between health-care providers and those who pay the bills for services, namely the government (for Medicare and Medicaid) and the insurance companies. At one time, physicians ordered whichever tests they felt necessary to diagnose problems and whichever treatments they deemed necessary to fix those problems. If a physician felt that a patient would benefit from an extra day in the hospital, the patient stayed in the hospital. If the physician ordered certain medications to treat the patient's problem, the patient received them. Now, physicians have been forced to use criteria established by insurance companies and the government for diagnosing, treating, admitting, and discharging patients—or the bill is not paid. In essence, the view of the insurance company and government is that physicians are free to treat patients as they deem necessary. However, if physicians deviate from the established standards and criteria for treatment, they are not paid. You may recall that, a few years ago, the standard used by those paying the bills was that patients were required to leave the hospital 24 hours after vaginal childbirth. The outcry from the public and from health-care providers grew so loud that the length of stay for vaginal delivery has now increased to 48 hours. But 20 years ago, a woman stayed in the hospital for 4 or 5 days after such a delivery.

Although this is a simple explanation of the current state of affairs regarding payment for services and maintaining quality of care, it is a very complex problem. The complexity exists because the government and insurance agencies differ in types of payment plans and criteria that form the standards of care. In addition, the criteria are under constant revision.

### ▄ Utilization Review Standards

Documentation of detailed assessments, accuracy of diagnoses, and appropriateness of treatments and follow-up are constantly being reviewed in all health-care settings (such as private physicians' offices, outpatient facilities, or hospitals). Everything and everyone is under the utilization review, which is the process of evaluating care given by nurses and physicians and all other health-care providers and agencies. Nurses primarily manage the utilization reviews, armed with specific criteria for auditing individual health-care providers and the delivery of services in each health-care setting. These nurses are hired by health-care agencies and by insurance companies. Utilization reviewers do not usually have direct contact with patients; they only re- view charts. They judge the necessity and appropriateness of care and the efficiency with which care is delivered.

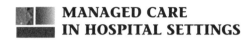

## MANAGED CARE IN HOSPITAL SETTINGS

There is a direct relationship between the care standards described above and the management of care. Currently, nearly all patients who enter hospitals find themselves in managed care delivery systems. Typically, patients entering health-care facilities have nurse case managers assigned to monitor and coordinate their progress through the health-care system. These case managers are experienced nurses, with most holding advanced degrees or specialty certifications. These nurses carefully manage hospital resources and coordinate discharge planning. With strict criteria imposed by government and insurance agencies to ensure rapid discharge from acute-care facilities, all nurses must carefully document and justify complications and additional problems with patients to ensure that quality care is rendered and financial obligations are met (that is, the bills are paid by government and insurance agencies). These nurses monitor patient progress, and especially track high-risk patients, as well as all patients with complications. These hospital-based nurse case managers interact with service providers and with insurance providers; thus, they are considered resource managers. It is essential to make links for patients to home health services, transitional care units, long-term care facilities, and other agencies to provide quality care.

## CHAPTER SUMMARY

The purpose of concept map care planning is to assist with critical thinking, analysis of clinical data, and planning comprehensive nursing care for your patients. A concept map is based on theories of learning and educational psychology, and is a diagrammatic teaching/learning strategy that provides you with the opportunity to visualize interrelationships between medical and nursing diagnoses, assessment data, and treatments. These visual maps and interventions are personal pocket guides to patient care, and they form the basis for discussion of nursing care between you and your clinical faculty.

Before developing a concept map, you must perform a comprehensive patient assessment. Then, in Step 1 of concept mapping, you develop a skeleton diagram of health problems. In Step 2, you analyze and categorize specific patient assessment data. In Step 3, you indicate relationships between nursing and medical diagnoses. In Step 4, you develop patient goals, outcomes, and nursing interventions for each nursing diagnosis. And in Step 5, you evaluate the patient's response to each specific nursing intervention and summarize your clinical impressions.

The development of concept map care planning is based on understanding and integrating accepted standards of patient care. Standards of care are derived from the standards of the ANA, the JCAHO, standard nursing care plans, standards of patient teaching, clinical pathways, insurance agency and government payment standards, and utilization review standards. As a result of these standards, hospitals have become centers for managed care and are employing nursing case managers as patient care resource coordinators. All parties involved with health-care delivery, including health-care agencies, health-care providers, insurance companies, and the government are finding ways to decrease costs while attempting to maintain quality services through managed care.

## LEARNING ACTIVITIES

1. Identify the names and locations of books and computer software that contain standardized nursing care plans that you can use as standards for patient care.
2. Locate samples of standards of care at your assigned clinical agency. Bring to class for discussion a standard nursing care plan from a local agency, a clinical pathway, a standardized specific procedure, and patient education materials.
3. Locate the procedure manual from a local health-care agency and compare a procedure you are currently learning from your procedures text to the same procedure in the agency's manual.
4. Identify the person or people at your agency who perform case management, discharge planning, and utilization review. Invite one of them to a clinical postconference to describe their role in decreasing costs while maintaining quality of care in the managed care environment.

## REFERENCES

1. Novak, J, and Gowin, DB: Learning How to Learn. Cambridge University Press, New York, 1984.
2. Ausubel, DP, Novak, JD, and Hanesian, H: Educational Psychology: A Cognitive View, ed 2. Werbel and Peck, New York, 1986.
3. Worrell, P: Metacognition: Implications for instruction in nursing education. J Nurs Educ 29(4):170, 1990.
4. All, AC, and Havens, RL: Cognitive/concept map: A teaching strategy for nursing. J Adv Nurs 25:1210, 1997.
5. Baugh, NG, and Mellott, KG: Clinical concept maps as preparation for student nurses' clinical experiences. J Nurs Educ 37(6):253, 1998.
6. Daley, BJ, et al: Concept maps: A strategy to teach and evaluate critical thinking. J Nurs Educ 38(1):42, 1999.
7. Daley, B: Concept maps: Linking nursing theory to clinical nursing practice. Journal of Continuing Education in Nursing 27(1):17, 1996.
8. Irvine, L: Can concept maps be used to promote meaningful learning in nurse education? J Adv Nurs 21:1175, 1995.
9. Kathol, DD, et al: Clinical correlation map: A tool for linking theory and practice. Nurse Educator. 23(4):31, 1998.
10. Novak, J, and Gowin, DB: Op cit.
11. Ausubel, DP, et al: Op cit.
12. American Philosophical Association. Critical thinking: A statement of expert consensus for purposes

of educational assessment and instruction. Center on Education and Training for Employment, College of Education, The Ohio State University. (ERIC Document Reproduction No. ED 315-423) Columbus, Ohio, 1990.

13. Schuster, PM: Concept maps: Reducing clinical care plan paperwork and increasing learning. Nurse Educator. 25(2):76, 2000.

14. Nursing's social policy statement. American Nurses Association, Washington, D.C., 1995.

15. Standards of Clinical Nursing Practice, ed 2. American Nurses Publishing, American Nurses Foundation/American Nurses Association, Washington, D.C., 1998.

16. Schuster, PM: Op cit.

17. Ibid.

18. Ibid.

19. Ibid.

20. Standards of Clinical Nursing Practice, ed 2., Op cit.

# Chapter 2

## Gathering Clinical Data:
### The Framework for Concept Map Care Plans

### O B J E C T I V E S

1. Identify nursing standards of care for systematically gathering clinical data to construct a basic patient profile database.

2. Describe essential components of a basic patient profile database that are needed to develop a concept map care plan.

3. Explain the purpose of each component of the basic patient profile database.

4. Identify where to search for clinical data in health-care agencies to develop basic patient profile databases.

5. Identify standardized forms to obtain from the agency relevant to concept map care planning.

6. Describe how to communicate with staff in the agency when you cannot find clinical data.

Gathering assessment data is the most important thing that student nurses do. This is because each decision regarding patient care is based on clinical data. Sound clinical judgments are based on accurate and complete data collection. The best nurses are excellent at assessment and know why each piece of assessment data is important to the clinical picture.

Many nursing students feel overwhelmed trying to collect relevant clinical data for their first patient assignments when they arrive at a new clinical unit or agency. These same feelings occur each time the student moves to a new agency. As a matter of fact, even experienced nurses feel intimidated by moving from a familiar agency or unit to a new clinical setting, because they fear they may miss important symptoms that will hinder their ability to make sound clinical judgments.

The purpose of this chapter is to give you guidelines for collecting relevant clinical data based on standards of nursing care. Nursing students are sometimes confused about what is and what is not important clinical data. Therefore, the chapter will describe the reasons why each piece of data is needed, along with where to look for the information you need to develop a plan of care. In addition, the chapter outlines the important skill of communicating effectively with staff when you cannot find the information you need to develop a plan of care.

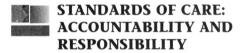

## STANDARDS OF CARE: ACCOUNTABILITY AND RESPONSIBILITY

Nursing students learn early in their nursing programs that they must be accountable and responsible. That is, student nurses are responsible for the nursing care they administer to their assigned patients. Student nurses must account for their clinical performance to clinical faculty, who are responsible and accountable for each student. In a clinical agency, the faculty accounts primarily to the nursing manager regarding student activities related to caring for patients. The nurse manager oversees the provision of nursing care.

In addition to being accountable to their faculty, students work directly with agency staff nurses and are also accountable to them. Agency nurses are responsible for overseeing the care of your patients, and they report directly to the nursing manager. You must know who the staff nurse is for your patient at all times and keep this nurse and your clinical faculty informed of current assessment information. You must tell this nurse the interventions you will and will not be able to provide to the patient. You must never leave patients for a break or any other reason without giving the staff nurses and your clinical faculty the most recent assessment data for your assigned patients. Communication between you, your faculty, and the cover nurse is critical for safe nursing care of patients.

Student nurses, clinical faculty, and the nursing staff at each agency are legally responsible and accountable. Professional nurses and student nurses may be taken to court and prosecuted for acting in an irresponsible manner. This may sound threatening, but professional nurses and student nurses are responsible and accountable

for the care of human beings. Nursing care of patients involves awesome responsibility with legal consequences for acting irresponsibly.

Standards of care are inextricably linked to professional accountability and responsibility. You, your faculty, and staff nurses must follow standards of care to act accountably and responsibly. The American Nurses Association (ANA) first standard of practice will be the focus of this chapter. This standard involves the collection of data. Specifically, the ANA states that collection of data about a patient's health status is to be systematic and continuous, and that data must be accessible, recorded, and communicated.[1] The Joint Commission on Accreditation of Healthcare Organizations (JCAHO) also upholds this same standard.

Data collection occurs *before* development of a plan of care, *before* implementation of nursing care, *during* implementation of nursing care, and *during* evaluation of the patient; therefore it is continuous. All of the data must be written down on patient records and be accessible to all healthcare providers. The frustrating problem for many students is that they do not know where to look for data in a clinical area. What's more, especially early in their nursing education, students typically do not know the most important data to collect. Sometimes students cannot read the writing or understand the abbreviations. Keep in mind that the data is there somewhere; you just have to find it! According to ANA standard 1, data must be accessible and recorded. Once you have found the data, of course, you have to know what it means and why it is important.

## FINDING IMPORTANT DATA

Students are usually given course assessment guidelines to follow when collecting data on patients. A typical example of a database patient profile is found in Figure 2–1. This basic patient profile database has been used to collect data for patients admitted to inpatient or outpatient agencies such as hospitals or outpatient same-day surgical centers. This assessment tool will serve as the basis of the concept map to be discussed in Chapter 3.

# PATIENT PROFILE DATABASE

## ADMISSION INFORMATION

Student Name ..............................................................................

| ❶ Date of Care: | ❷ Patient Initials: | ❸ Age:<br>(face sheet) | ❸ Growth and Development: | ❹ Sex:<br>(face sheet) | ❺ Admission Date:<br>(face sheet) |
|---|---|---|---|---|---|

**❻ Reason for Hospitalization** (face sheet):

**❼ Medical Diagnoses:** (present diagnoses, past diagnoses; physician's History and Physical notes in chart; nursing intake assessment and Kardex)

**❽ Surgical Procedures** (consent forms and Kardex):

## ❾ ADVANCE DIRECTIVES (NURSE'S ADMISSION ASSESSMENTS):

Living will: ☐ yes ☐ no      Power of attorney: ☐ yes ☐ no      Do not resuscitate (DNR) order (Kardex): ☐ yes ☐ no

## ❿ LABORATORY DATA

| Test | Norms | On admission | Current value | Test | Norms | On admission | Current value |
|---|---|---|---|---|---|---|---|
| White blood cells | | | | Potassium | | | |
| Differential | | | | Blood Glucose | | | |
| Hemoglobin | | | | Glycohemoglobin | | | |
| Hematocrit | | | | Cholesterol | | | |
| Platelets | | | | Low-density lipoproteins | | | |
| Prothrombin time | | | | Urine analysis | | | |
| International normalized ratio | | | | | | | |
| Activated partial thromboplastin time | | | | Other abnormal | | | |

## ⑪ DIAGNOSTIC TESTS

| Chest x-ray: | EKG: | Other abnormal reports: |
|---|---|---|
| Other: | Other: | Other: |

## ⑫ MEDICATIONS

*List medications and times of administration (medication administration record and check the drawer in the carts for spelling):*

| Medication/Time of Administration | Medication/Time of Administration | Medication/Time of Administration |
|---|---|---|
| | | |
| | | |
| | | |
| | | |
| | | |
| | | |

■ *Figure* 2–1

Patient profile database.

*(Continued)*

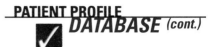
## ALLERGIES / PAIN

**13** Allergies (medication administration records):

**14** When was the last pain medication given? (medication administration record):

**14** Where is the pain? (nurse's notes):

**14** How much pain is the patient in on a scale from 0 – 10? (nurse's notes, flow sheet):

## TREATMENTS

**15** Treatments (Kardex):

**16** Support services (Kardex):

**17** Consultations (Kardex):

## 18 DIET / FLUIDS

| Type of Diet (Kardex): | Restrictions (Kardex): | Gag reflex intact:<br>☐ yes ☐ no | Appetite: | Breakfast<br>_____ % | Lunch<br>_____ % | Supper<br>_____ % |
|---|---|---|---|---|---|---|

*Circle Those Problems That Apply:*

Fluid intake:
24 hours
(flow sheet)

Tube feedings:
type and rate
(Kardex)

- Problems: swallowing, chewing, dentures (nurse's notes)
- Needs assistance with feeding (nurse's notes)
- Nausea or vomiting (nurse's notes)
- Overhydrated or dehydrated (evaluate total intake and output on flow sheet)
- Belching          • Other: _____

## 19 INTRAVENOUS FLUIDS (IV therapy record)

| Type and rate: | IV dressing dry, no edema, redness of site:<br>☐ yes ☐ no | Other: |
|---|---|---|

## 20 ELIMINATION (flow sheet)

| Last bowel movement: | 24-hour urine output: | Foley/condom catheter:<br>☐ yes ☐ no |
|---|---|---|

*Circle Those Problems That Apply:*

- Bowel:      constipation      diarrhea      flatus      incontinence      belching
- Urinary:      hesitancy      frequency      burning      incontinence      odor
- Other: _____

## 21 ACTIVITY (Kardex, flow sheet)

| Ability to walk (gait): | Type of activity orders: | Use of assistive devices: cane, walker, crutches, prosthesis: | Falls-risk assessment rating: |
|---|---|---|---|

| No. of side rails required (flow sheet): | Restraints (flow sheet):<br>☐ yes ☐ no | Weakness:<br>☐ yes ☐ no | Trouble sleeping (nurse's notes):<br>☐ yes ☐ no |
|---|---|---|---|

## PHYSICAL ASSESSMENT DATA

| **22** BP (flow sheet): | **22** TPR (flow sheet): | **23**<br>Height: _____    Weight: _____    (nursing intake assessments) |
|---|---|---|

■ *Figure* **2–1** (continued)

**REVIEW OF SYSTEMS** *Write WNL (within normal limits) if normal and describe abnormalities in space provided: (check nurses' notes and shift assessments for the latest information you can get)*

**PATIENT PROFILE**
✓ *DATABASE (cont.)*

**24  NEUROLOGICAL/MENTAL STATUS:** _____

| LOC: alert and oriented to person, place, time (A&O x 3) confused, etc. | Speech: clear, appropriate/inappropriate |
|---|---|

| Motor: ROM x 4 extremities | Sensation: 4 extremities | Pupils: PERRLA | Sensory deficits for vision/hearing/taste/smell |
|---|---|---|---|

**25  MUSCULOSKELETAL SYSTEM:** _____

| Bones, joints, muscles (fractures, contractures, arthritis, spinal curvatures, etc.): | Extremity circulation checks (pulses, temperature, sensation, edema): |
|---|---|
| Ted hose/plexi pulses/compression devices: type: | Casts, splint, collar, brace: |

**26  CARDIOVASCULAR SYSTEM:** _____

| Pulses (radial, pedal) (to touch or with Doppler): | Capillary refill (<3 s): ☐ yes ☐ no | Edema, pitting vs. nonpitting: |
|---|---|---|
| Neck vein (distention): | Sounds: $S_1$, $S_2$, regular, irregular: | Any chest pain: |

**27  RESPIRATORY SYSTEM:** _____

| Depth, rate, rhythm: | Use of accessory muscles: | Cyanosis: | Sputum: color, amount: | Cough: productive, nonproductive: | Breath sounds: clear, rales, wheezes: |
|---|---|---|---|---|---|
| Use of oxygen: nasal cannula, mask, trach collar: | Flow rate of oxygen: | Oxygen humidification: ☐ yes ☐ no | Pulse oximeter: _____ % oxygen saturation | | Smoking: ☐ yes ☐ no |

**28  GASTROINTESTINAL SYSTEM:** _____

| Abdominal pain, tenderness, guarding; distention, soft, firm: | Bowel sounds x 4 quadrants: | NG tube: describe drainage: |
|---|---|---|
| Ostomy: describe stoma site and stools: | Other: | |

**29  SKIN AND WOUNDS:** _____

| Color, turgor: | Rash, bruises: | Describe wounds (size, location): | Edges approximated: ☐ yes ☐ no | Type of wound drains: |
|---|---|---|---|---|
| Characteristics of drainage: | Dressings (clean, dry, intact): | Sutures, staples, steri-strips, other: | Risk for decubitus ulcer assessment rating: | Other: |

**30  EYES, EARS, NOSE, THROAT (EENT):** _____

| Eyes: redness, drainage, edema, ptosis | Ears: drainage | Nose: redness, drainage, edema | Throat: sore |
|---|---|---|---|

**PSYCHOSOCIAL AND CULTURAL ASSESSMENT:**

| 31 Religious preference (face sheet): | 32 Marital status (face sheet): | 33 Health-care benefits and insurance (face sheet): | 34 Occupation (face sheet): | 35 Emotional state (nurse's notes): |
|---|---|---|---|---|

**Additional information to obtain from clinical units the night before clinical specific to your patient's diagnosis:**

| Standardized falls-risk assessment: ☐ yes ☐ no | Pressure ulcer assessment: ☐ yes ☐ no | Standardized skin assessment: ☐ yes ☐ no | Standardized nursing care plans: ☐ yes ☐ no | Clinical pathways: ☐ yes ☐ no | Patient education materials: ☐ yes ☐ no |
|---|---|---|---|---|---|

■ *Figure* **2–1** *(continued)*

You must know the essential components of a basic patient profile database, the purpose of each component of the profile, and where to search for the information in health-care agencies. This database has physical, psychological, social, and cultural components. Ninety-nine percent of it is collected from patient notes and records, whereas one percent may be collected from a brief encounter with your patient and a conversation with the patient's assigned agency nurse. It is best if you can obtain your assignment the evening before clinical, because you have more time to think critically and analyze the data you obtained and put together a care plan. In outpatient settings, this may not be possible. Students who are unable to obtain an assignment the day before clinical may have to collect data and develop a care plan on the day of care. Each component of the database will be described carefully in the following sections. Refer to Figure 2–1 as you read the remainder of the chapter. Each component of the patient database in Figure 2–1 has been numbered to correspond with the explanations for each component written in the following sections.

## 1. Student Name and Date of Care

Your name and date of care are needed to help your clinical faculty keep your database separate from those of the other nursing students at your clinical agency.

## 2. Patient Initials

Never write a patient's full name on anything that will be taken out of the hospital. All information recorded on the patient profile is confidential. Confidentiality involves ethical and legal standards of care. It is your ethical and legal responsibility to reveal confidential information only to health-care professionals directly involved in the patient's care. Be very careful what you do with confidential information. Never leave forms lying around in patient rooms where the patient, family, and friends may read what you have written, even if you include only initials on the data. Never discuss data with anyone outside the health-care agency.

If a patient's family or friends ask a general question about how the patient is doing, give a general answer, such as, "Fine. He's coming along nicely. He ate well and he's up and moving around" or, "Not so good today. He's hurting and tired." However, do not reveal the specifics of the diagnosis and prognosis. You should tell the inquiring person that the information is confidential and that he should discuss the specifics directly with the patient or with the physician.

## 3. Age, Growth, and Development

The patient's age can be obtained from the face sheet of the chart. It is one of the first few sheets that you will find as you open the chart. The face sheet is the page that is typed by the hospital registration department. On entry to the health-care agency, the first stop the patient makes is the registration desk where the patient (or a family member) registers for admission.

Age is a very important factor to consider as you prepare for your assignment. You must be aware of the human growth and developmental tasks across the life span, and then consider how the current health problem has affected the patient's ability to accomplish the developmental tasks at hand. Eric H. Erickson[2] has a widely known theory of eight stages of human growth and development with which you should be familiar.

### STAGE 1: TRUST VERSUS MISTRUST

During the first year of life, an infant must learn to trust the people in his environment. When caretakers meet the infant's needs for food, warmth, security, and love, the infant will learn to expect what will happen and can trust those around him to provide for what he needs. He feels secure. When an infant's needs are not met, he becomes fearful and mistrusting. Some of these infants fail to thrive. Failure to thrive is a medical diagnosis in which an infant may fail to gain weight or may even lose it. This problem may stem from such environmental causes as physical starvation or emotional deprivation of love and security.

### STAGE 2: AUTONOMY VERSUS SHAME AND DOUBT

During the first few years of life, about ages 1 to 3, children explore their surroundings and gain increasing autonomy from their caretakers. The toddler needs lots of support and encouragement to learn to walk and control bowel and bladder functioning. If parents belittle the toddler, self-doubt and shame occur, and a sense of inferiority may take root.

## STAGE 3: INITIATIVE VERSUS GUILT

From about ages 3 to 6, children begin to manipulate their environments and become very active. As they take on new challenges successfully with parental support and encouragement, children learn to take the initiative. Lack of parental support and inappropriate scolding for attempts to try new things may lead to feelings of resentment and unworthiness.

## STAGE 4: INDUSTRY VERSUS INFERIORITY

A new stage begins as the child enters school and lasts until puberty. Children must learn a new set of social rules as they enter school and develop roles and relationships with teachers and peers outside of their family. Throughout this stage, they must learn to be productive workers at school and at home. Children are expected to develop many self-care skills. They are gradually becoming independent of their families and learning about self-sufficiency. Without parental support, encouragement, and guidance, children may feel inferior and inadequate, and they may lose faith in their own ability to become self-sufficient.

## STAGE 5: EGO IDENTITY VERSUS ROLE DIFFUSION

The adolescent is searching for personal identity. Establishing identity involves successful integration of many social roles, such as student, sibling, friend, cheerleader, athlete, band member, or key club member. These roles must form coherent patterns that give young people a sense of who they are—their identities. Adolescents need to form close relationships with peers and develop a sexual identity. Their value systems are evolving. They must learn to appreciate their achievements and, toward the end of this stage, select a career. Failure to accomplish this may lead to feelings of hopelessness, despair, and confusion.

## STAGE 6: INTIMACY VERSUS ISOLATION

The primary task of young adulthood is to love someone else, to form an intimate bond with an-other person. Failure to accomplish intimacy leads to loneliness. Important tasks include maintaining friendships and establishing new social groups while taking on civic responsibilities in communities. In addition, young adults have the task of growing independent from their parents' home and managing their own households. To do so, they must establish a career. Many choose to marry. Many have their own children and take on parenting roles, which include encouraging and supporting their own children as those children attempt to accomplish the growth and developmental tasks already discussed. In addition, young adults are in the process of formulating a meaningful philosophy of life.

## STAGE 7: GENERATIVITY VERSUS STAGNATION

During middle adulthood, the challenge is to remain productive and creative in all aspects of life and to find meaning and joy in careers, family, and community social participation. In contrast to feelings of generativity are feelings of stagnation. Life may become a boring routine, and a person may feel resentful when tasks of this stage are not successfully accomplished. To successfully accomplish this stage of life, individuals may need to review and redirect goals to achieve desired performance in a career. They also may need to develop satisfying hobby and leisure activities.

Middle adults must also accept and adjust to the physical changes of middle age, such as wearing glasses, getting wrinkles, and seeing gray hair. In addition, they need to make adjustments in lifestyles to accommodate aging parents and to maintain relationships with their mates. Those with adolescent children need to assist them in searching for identity and then, as the children leave home, cope with an "empty nest" feeling. As children leave, relationships with spouses are redefined. There may be new roles of in-law and grandparent by the end of this stage.

## STAGE 8: EGO INTEGRITY VERSUS DESPAIR

During late adulthood, those with a sense of ego integrity have attained an acceptance of their lives and feelings that life has been complete and satisfactory. During this stage, individuals conduct life reviews, in which they consider their successes and failures and prepare for the inevitability of death. The task is to make peace with one's self. Although the person may not have accomplished everything that she had hoped, she reconciles that it is an imperfect world, and she did the best she could, given the set of circumstances in her life. She faces death without fear, content that she has played a meaningful part in the lives of those around her. In addition, the person must continue to affiliate with others the same age, while adjusting to the death of friends, family members, and spouse.

In contrast to ego integrity is despair. Those in despair believe that too much wrong has occurred and that there is no time to make things better. They may be filled with feelings of resentment, futility, hopelessness, and fear of death.

During this time period, the tasks also include adjusting to changes in physical strength and health, and arranging satisfactory physical living quarters. This includes maintaining a home or apartment, or moving to a retirement center or nursing home. With retirement from the workforce, there is an adjustment to retirement and reduced income. With the loss of work roles, the person must find activities that enhance self-worth and usefulness. Some people feel free to pursue whatever activities are important to them. These activities may include a "semi-retired" career, a hobby, a sport, or community service activities.

### RELEVANCE OF GROWTH AND DEVELOPMENT TO HEALTH STATE

These eight stages and their associated tasks should be foremost on your mind when you think about your patient's age. A key question is the effect a health problem and its treatment is having and will have on the person's ability to pursue the tasks of a particular age. You can assume that a person's life work has been at least temporarily altered. Depending on the health problem involved, the course of the person's life may be altered permanently. You can also assume that all people entering a health-care setting would rather be doing their life's work and accomplishing the tasks of their age instead of working with you and the other health-care providers. The challenge to nurses is to get patients back on track and to promote optimal lev-

els of growth and development or a peaceful death.

### ■ 4. Sex

Look at the face sheet to find the patient's sex. It is important that you be aware of gender differences in communication and that you communicate clearly with both sexes. Specifically, women tend to be focused on affiliation through communication, wanting to establish intimacy and forming communal connections. In contrast, men tend to be focused on attaining independence and status through communication, and are concerned with hierarchy in human relationships. These differing gender goals influence the nature of human relationships, including the relationships between health-care providers and patients. So for example, to some men, illness may be viewed as taking away independence and status, resulting in feelings of powerlessness. In contrast, women who are functioning with affiliative goals in mind may willingly accept the support provided by health-care providers. As you perform assessments, be aware of gender differences in communication so that you can clearly decipher messages from both sexes.[3,4]

### ■ 5. Admission Date

Look to the face sheet for this information as well. It is important to know how long the person has been in the health-care system. With managed care, there is usually a specific amount of time allotted to each type of problem. For example, a patient having knee replacement is in the hospital for 3 to 4 days. You can begin to determine if your patient is on or off the expected course of treatment just by knowing the date of admission and the expected length of stay for the type of problem for which the patient was admitted.

### ■ 6. Reason for Hospitalization

Again, the face sheet has this information. The reason for hospitalization is typed clearly on the face sheet without abbreviations. Many students struggle with abbreviations and poor handwriting, both of which can be avoided by obtaining the reason for hospitalization from the face sheet. This is generally a medical diagnosis and, if applicable, includes the surgical procedure. Although many things may have happened to a patient during hospitalization, it is important to know what the initial problem was that brought the person into the hospital in the first place.

## ▰ 7. Medical Diagnoses

The face sheet contains information on present and past medical diagnoses in addition to the reason for hospitalization. It is important to note the current medical diagnoses as well as previous medical diagnoses. This information on medical diagnoses is also found on the nurse's initial intake history and physical assessment forms, and the physician's history and physical assessment forms. These are all located in the patient's chart. Many, but not all, facilities summarize pertinent information on a Kardex. The Kardex is a quick reference for nurses that contains critical information for the most current care of the patient. Facilities that use a Kardex may have slight variations in format; however, the information contained on it is almost universal.

When you get home, you must look up each medical diagnosis in your pathophysiology book, which will have the most complete definition with pathological effects and the etiology of the disease. It is not at all uncommon for the same patient to have a number of diagnoses. For example, a patient may have a history of diabetes and hypertension but is currently being admitted for a small bowel obstruction. All medical problems must be identified and defined because you must have a clear picture of the clinical problems to develop the nursing care plan.

## ▰ 8. Surgical Procedures

The best place to find out what types of surgical procedures the patient underwent (or is about to undergo) is on the surgical consent forms in the patient's chart. This is because legal standards demand that the exact procedure be specified and that no abbreviations are used. The surgical procedure is also listed on the Kardex. However, it is commonly abbreviated on the Kardex and therefore more difficult to interpret.

When defining surgical procedures, you can start with a medical dictionary for a basic definition. However the best reference is a nursing medical-surgical text with a more detailed description of the surgical procedure. Sometimes you can find typed surgical operative notes dictated by the surgeon and transcribed by people in the medical records department, but this is not usually available in the chart until a few days after surgery.

## ▰ 9. Advance Directives

This information is found on the admission nurse's assessment form; it should also appear on the Kardex. Health-care facilities are required by law to ask patients if they have advance directives. Advance directives are legal documents such as a living will and a health-care power of attorney. A living will outlines the patient's wishes about life-sustaining treatments; typically, it tells health-care providers to withhold life-sustaining treatments if the patient is in a terminal condition and cannot make his own decisions. A health-care power of attorney appoints a person to make health-care decisions on the patient's behalf if the patient is unable to do so.

DNR is a crucial abbreviation to remember. It stands for *do not resuscitate*. If the patient has a DNR order, it will be listed on the Kardex and sometimes with a red label on the outside of the chart. It means that the person does not want CPR if he goes into cardiac or respiratory arrest. The person may be given drugs and kept comfortable, but death is expected soon and a peaceful death with dignity is the goal.

## ▰ 10. Laboratory Values

A specific section of the chart is set aside for the patient's laboratory values.[5] Results of the blood and urine tests described in the following sections are important to know for any patient, whether the values are normal or abnormal. Many additional tests may be ordered based on the pathophysiology of the patient's disease. Of course, all currently abnormal results are very important because they reveal the extent of disease.

Make sure you know which tests are ordered for your clinical day of care because intravenous fluids and medication administration are directly linked to what is happening in the patient's blood and urine. You must check the new daily laboratory values before giving intravenous fluids and medications. For example, if you are giving insulin at 8 A.M., make sure you know the blood glucose value from the 6 A.M. draw. If the blood glucose is too low, the insulin may be held. Likewise, if you are giving Lovenox (enoxaparin sodium) at 8 A.M., make sure you know results of the patient's platelet test before you give the medication. The dose of Lovenox will be held if platelets drop too low.

You should know the values of your patient's blood for the following commonly ordered blood and urine tests. These tests are universally ordered on almost all patients and serve as a baseline assessment for planning nursing care.

## WHITE BLOOD CELLS

The abbreviation for white blood cells is WBCs. As a rule of thumb, the WBC count should be less than 10,000/mm³. An elevation of WBCs indicates inflammation and infection. The WBCs may be broken down into a differential count of each cell type. An increase in the number of neutrophils (band and stab cells) indicate an acute infection, also known as a "shift to the left." Other types of WBCs (basophils and eosinophils) are elevated in allergic reactions. Still others (lymphocytes) are involved with developing immunity and phagocytic monocytes that engulf bacteria. A low WBC count (below 5,000/mm³) indicates problems in producing cells from the bone marrow, which may accompany chemotherapy.

## HEMOGLOBIN AND HEMATOCRIT

These are commonly abbreviated as H&H or Hgb & Hct. Hemoglobin is a reflection of the amount of red blood cells in the blood, usually 14 to 18 g/dL in male patients and 12 to 16 g/dL in female patients. The main reason that the hemoglobin level drops is bleeding. When the hemoglobin level drops below 9 g/dL, blood transfusions may be required. A commonly used term for low hemoglobin is anemia. In addition to blood loss, anemia may be the result of poor nutrition (in addition to many other causes).

Hematocrit is the percentage of red blood cells in the total blood volume. The total blood volume is composed of red blood cells and serum. In male patients, a normal hematocrit is 42% to 52%. In female patients, a normal hematocrit is 37% to 47%. The hematocrit should be about three times the Hgb concentration. When the patient is bleeding, hematocrit will drop along with the hemoglobin level. Hematocrit also reflects the patient's state of hydration. Sometimes the hemoglobin level is normal or slightly high and the hematocrit is low. This occurs when the patient is dehydrated.

## BLOOD COAGULATION STUDIES

These studies include platelet counts and international normalized ratio (INR), prothrombin time (PT), partial thromboplastin time (PTT), and activated partial thromboplastin time (aPTT).

### Platelets

Platelets are thrombocytes, which are cells essential to blood clotting. Normal platelet counts are between 150,000 to 400,000/mm³. In addition to bleeding, platelets typically decrease because certain drugs can hinder the bone marrow from producing these cells. For example, Lovenox (enoxaparin), which is used to prevent formation of blood clots in the legs in immobilized patients, has the side effect of decreasing platelets. For that reason, platelet counts are monitored during Lovenox administration. The drug is usually discontinued when platelets drop below 130,000/mm³.

### INR, PT, PTT, and aPTT

Values for INR, PT (sometimes called "pro time"), PTT, and aPTT reflect different ways to express the time it takes for blood to coagulate and clot. The therapeutic INR level for treatment has a range of 2.0 to 3.0. The PT is normally 11 to 12.5 seconds. PTT is normally 60 to 70 seconds. And aPTT is normally 30 to 40 seconds. Although these values all reflect blood-clotting ability, they differ somewhat: PTT or aPTT is used to assess the intrinsic system of clotting, and PT or INR is used to assess the extrinsic system of clotting. These values are very important because many patients take anticoagulants to increase the time it takes for a clot to form. For example, immobilized patients are routinely placed on anticoagulation therapy to prevent formation of blood clots.

The PTT (aPTT) is used to assess the effects of the anticoagulant heparin, which is given subcutaneously or intravenously. The PT or INR is used to assess the effect of the anticoagulant Coumadin (warfarin), which is given orally. Heparin affects the intrinsic system of clotting, and Coumadin affects the extrinsic system of clotting.

In either case, patients receiving anticoagulant therapy will have purposely prolonged clotting times that are 1.5 to 2.5 times the control value. Heparin and Coumadin dosages are regulated up or down to maintain the anticoagulation at 1.5 to 2.5 times the control value. Therefore, you must be sure to know the patient's latest INR or PT before giving Coumadin, the latest aPTT or PTT before giving heparin, or the latest platelet counts before giving Lovenox.

## ELECTROLYTES

Probably the most important electrolyte to be aware of is potassium. The normal potassium level is about 3.5 to 5.5 mEq/L. Too much or too little of this electrolyte will have profound effects on all muscles. However, the muscle of major concern for altered potassium levels is the heart muscle. The ability of the heart to contract and the rate at which it contracts both depend on normal potassium levels. Potassium levels typically decline with vomiting and diarrhea. Potassium-depleting diuretics are another common cause of decreased potassium levels.

Potassium is commonly added to intravenous fluids and given in oral preparations. Make sure you know the patient's latest potassium levels before giving potassium supplements, either intravenously or orally. In addition, patients taking Lanoxin (digitalis) may develop toxic levels of this drug in their bloodstream when potassium levels are too low, inducing serious cardiac arrhythmias.

## BLOOD GLUCOSE AND GLYCOSYLATED HEMOGLOBIN

These tests are used to assess a patient's current glucose level and long-term glucose control.

### Blood Glucose

The level of glucose in a patient's blood after fasting (also known as the fasting blood sugar) is normally 70 to 120 mg/dL of blood. Persistently elevated blood glucose levels may indicate diabetes mellitus. Because diabetes is so common, this is a common test.

Typically, when the blood glucose level is too low, the cause is unintentional insulin overdose. Consider this example: A patient's 6 A.M. glucose level is within normal limits, so the nurse gives the patient's 7 A.M. insulin thinking that he will be eating breakfast. But the patient begins feeling nauseated and doesn't eat. In this case, expect an insulin reaction because the blood glucose is guaranteed to drop.

Patients who are "brittle," which means that their blood glucose is not under control and can fluctuate widely, should be checked in the morning, usually around 6 A.M. The result of this test is the fasting blood glucose. Non-fasting blood glucose levels are commonly checked before lunch, before supper, and at bedtime. In brittle diabetics, insulin is given on a sliding scale based on the blood glucose readings (see Table 2–1).

### Glycosylated Hemoglobin

Glycosylated hemoglobin (also called glycohemoglobin) is another common test of blood glucose. It is used to measure long-term blood glucose control over a period of up to 120 days. Glucose binds to hemoglobin in a chemical reaction. When the patient is diabetic and blood glucose levels are elevated, the percentage of glycosylated hemoglobin is higher. This reaction is

| *Table 2-1* Sliding Scale Insulin Dosages | |
|---|---|
| The higher the blood glucose, the more insulin is needed to regulate blood glucose levels. Sample guidelines for regular sliding scale insulin are as follows: | |
| **BLOOD GLUCOSE LEVEL** | **INSULIN DOSAGE** |
| 151–200 mg/dL | 6 U |
| 201–250 mg/dL | 8 U |
| 251–300 mg/dL | 10 U |
| 301–400 mg/dL | 12 U |

not reversible; once the glycogen attaches, it remains with the red blood cell for its life cycle, about 120 days. Therefore, you can tell if the patient's blood glucose has been under control over a period of time. Normal healthy people have 5.5% to 8.8% of total hemoglobin bound to glucose. Diabetics under control range from 7.5% to 11.4% total hemoglobin bound to glucose, whereas those who need either more diet instruction or more insulin (or both) will be higher. There are actually three types of hemoglobin that become glycosylated: A1a, A1b, and A1c. Many laboratories report only the A1c level, which is normally 3.56% bound to glucose.[6]

## CHOLESTEROL

The cholesterol level indicates the amount of lipids or fats in the blood. Lipids are carried in the blood in combination with proteins, and are thus called lipoproteins. High levels of cholesterol are a risk factor for cardiovascular disease, which is the primary health problem in the United States. Numerous people have cholesterol levels above 200 mg/dL. Cholesterol is composed of high-density lipoproteins (HDLs), low-density lipoproteins (LDLs), and triglycerides.

Of primary interest in relation to cardiac disease are the LDLs, which should be less than 130 mg/dL. LDLs have been called "bad" cholesterol because they produce atherosclerosis. Many people take lipid-lowering drugs such as Lipitor (atorvastatin calcium) to reduce their LDL levels. They also are prescribed a low cholesterol diet and exercise program.

## URINE ANALYSIS AND CULTURE FOR BACTERIA

Urine testing is done mainly to check for infection and also to check kidney function. Bladder infections are extremely common, especially in women because they have a shorter urethra than men do. Typically, a clean catch urine specimen is obtained. The patient wipes the urethra with special antiseptic solution, voids a little in the toilet, and then inserts a sterile cup under the urine stream until the cup contains about 30 mL. This specimen should contain less than 10,000 bacteria/mL, provided the patient has wiped the urethra properly to decrease the number of normal flora around the meatus. A specimen obtained from a sterile catheterization, where a sterile tube is inserted into the sterile bladder, should contain no bacteria. In addition, the urine should contain no protein, blood, ketones, or glucose. Any of these substances in urine usually indicate diabetes or kidney disease.

Many other blood tests can be run as well. Other common blood tests include blood urea nitrogen (BUN) and creatinine levels to measure kidney function, bilirubin levels to measure liver function, and other electrolyte levels such as sodium, chloride, magnesium, phosphorus, and calcium. Always record any recent abnormal values (within 1 day of your clinical assignment), and record what the values were on admission.

## ■ 11. Diagnostic Tests

Your patient may undergo a wide range of diagnostic tests. Perhaps the two most common tests are a chest x-ray and an electrocardiogram (ECG).

### CHEST X-RAY

You can find chest x-ray reports in the patient's chart under laboratory and diagnostic procedures. The chest x-ray is a basic diagnostic test used to examine the structure of the heart and lungs. Enlargement of the heart and areas of lung consolidation, which could result from pneumonia or tumors, can be detected on chest x-rays.

### ECG

The ECG indicates patterns of electrical activity and contraction of the heart muscle. This test is routinely obtained on patients over age 35 as part of a general physical examination. This report is also found under laboratory and diagnostic procedures in the patient's chart. Although student nurses are not expected to interpret ECG tracings, the interpretation is printed on the report along with the rhythm strips indicating the rate and rhythm of the heart.

## ■ 12. Medications and Times of Administration

One of the most important and dangerous tasks for which nurses are responsible is medication administration. From virtually the first day of classes, nurses learn the six "rights" of drug administration:

- Right drug
- Right patient
- Right dose
- Right route
- Right time
- Right to refuse a medication

This sounds simple enough; yet, despite the best intentions of nurses and other health-care professionals, medication errors do occur. They can harm or even kill patients. Consequently, you must be exceedingly careful whenever you work with medications.

To find information about your patient's medications, look on the medication sheet, also known as the medication record, which usually is kept in the same place as the Kardex. List each drug and the times it should be administered on your patient profile database. Sometimes drugs are misspelled on these sheets. Therefore, you should go directly to the patients' medication drawer or wherever drugs are kept and copy the name and dosage of the drug from the paper wrapper on the drug. That way, you can be sure you have spelled the drug name correctly.

When you get home, you will need to look up and study each drug. You must know its actions and side effects, usual dosages, precautions, and what the patient should be taught about each drug. You may want to consider purchasing a set of drug cards so you can highlight important actions and side effects on the cards. Computer programs are also available for drug information, and they save time in finding information. Also consider looking on the Internet for drug information. Keep in mind that not every drug is available in any given drug reference.

If you are unable to find a drug in your reference books or computer programs at home, call the pharmacy at the health-care institution or the pharmacist at the local drugstore. Tell the pharmacist that you are a nursing student and would like information on a drug. For example, suppose you cannot find Alu-Tab tablets in your drug cards. Ask the pharmacist

to give you information about that drug over the phone.

As you research your drugs, always write down the trade name and the generic name of the drug. Many times the trade name is listed on a medication record, but a generic drug is substituted by the pharmacy. Sometimes, two generic drugs will be substituted for a single combination trade name drug. This may seem very confusing at first. For example, the trade name drug Diovan HCT contains both valsartan and hydrochlorothiazide in one tablet. The pharmacy may substitute two generic tablets: one tablet of valsartan and one tablet of hydrochlorothiazide. Substitutes are made by pharmacies to decrease the cost of brand name drugs. You must know the composition of each tablet to be administered, and you must be especially careful when combination drugs have been ordered.

It is most important to recognize the general classification to which any particular drug belongs. This will help you in identifying where the drug belongs on the concept map. For example:

- Antibiotics are grouped with the nursing diagnosis of **Risk for Infection**.
- Antidysrhythmics and antihypertensives are grouped with **Decreased Cardiac Output**.
- Anticoagulants and diuretics are grouped with **Deficient Fluid Volume**.
- Corticosteroids are grouped with **Ineffective Protection**.
- Anticonvulsants are grouped with **Ineffective Tissue Perfusion (cerebral)**.
- Insulins are grouped with **Imbalanced Nutrition: Less Than Body Requirements**.
- Drugs used for pain are grouped with **Acute Pain** or **Chronic Pain**.

## 13. Allergies

Allergies to drugs may appear in many places in patient records. Allergies to drugs are critical to note because an allergic reaction may lead to anaphylactic shock and death. In many institutions, the front of the chart itself will have a red label on it noting drug allergies. The medication record will have a space for drug allergies, and the Kardex will also list drug allergies.

## ■ 14. Pain Medications and Pain Ratings

Pain control is a task central to nursing care. Find out when the patient last received a pain medication, what type of medication it was, and the amount administered. You can find this information on the medication administration record. Also, look at the pattern of pain medication administration. This will give you an indication of the amount of pain the patient has been having. However, keep in mind that not all patients will ask for pain medication, even when they are uncomfortable.

### PAIN RATINGS

A patient's perception of pain is documented on the flow sheets and on the nursing notes. Patients are usually asked to rate the amount of pain they feel on a scale of 0 to 10, with 0 as no pain, and 10 as the worst pain ever experienced. You need to locate the most recent pain rating on the nursing notes. Subjective pain ratings can be used in addition to the data collected about the patient's use of pain medications to assess the pain. In addition, the nurses' notes will also indicate the location of the patient's pain.

## ■ 15. Treatments and Relation to Medical and Nursing Diagnoses

Examples of treatments include oxygen administration, incentive spirometry, catheters, nasogastric tubes, and dressing changes. They are all the things being done to the patient. You will eventually be responsible for ensuring that all treatments are done. The treatments are listed on the Kardex. It is important to note what these treatments are, even if you have not yet learned how to do them all. Your agency nurse may actually perform a treatment that you have not yet learned how to do.

Look up and define each treatment, and know why the patient is receiving the treatment as it relates to the medical and nursing diagnoses. For example, the patient may be instructed to do incentive spirometry breathing exercises every hour while awake to promote deep breathing and oxygenation in the lungs and to prevent pneumonia. When you make your map of major nursing diagnoses, this treatment will be grouped under the nursing diagnosis of **Impaired Gas Exchange**.

## ■ 16. Support Services

Support services are all the disciplines involved in the patient's care. These include physical therapy, occupational therapy, speech therapy, respiratory therapy, and social work. It is important to identify the role of each discipline in the patient's care. The nurse's role is to assess the patient's physical status and to recognize whether the patient will be able to tolerate the services that are scheduled. The nurse then communicates as appropriate with the support services and the attending physician, and gives recommendations for therapy.

For example, say the patient is supposed to be ambulated in the hall postoperatively after a total hip replacement. You know the patient's morning hemoglobin was 8 g/dL, she is scheduled for a transfusion, her blood pressure was lower than it was yesterday, her face is pale, and her nail beds are white. You are responsible for discussing patient data with the physical therapist and recommending that the patient be exercised in bed and ambulated to a chair, and that the physical therapist should wait until after the transfusion to get the patient up and walking in the hall.

In another example, the patient has asthma and receives inhalation treatments every 4 hours. You note that the patient's breathing is worsening even though the 4 hours aren't quite up yet. You should intervene and call the respiratory therapist to report the problem and ask if the therapist could arrive right on time or even a few minutes early for the next treatment.

## ■ 17. Consultations

Consultants are physicians who are specialists, such as cardiologists, pulmonologists, and gastroenterologists. They are also listed on the Kardex in the patient's chart. The primary doctor who admitted the patient to the hospital will call in a specialist when he or she suspects that the patient's medical problem resides in a specific organ system. In essence, the primary doctor is asking the opinion and treatment advice of the specialist. If you know the specialty of the consultants, you know which physiological components of the body to assess most carefully, because the primary physician would not need the services of the consultant unless something was likely to be wrong with that system of the body. Consultants typically focus on one body system.

### ■■ 18. Type of Diet

The type of diet the patient is following and any dietary restrictions are always listed on the Kardex. The nursing diagnosis **Imbalanced Nutrition** is very common, and patients often have knowledge deficits and problems in managing and adhering to prescribed diets. A regular or general diet is based on the food pyramid guidelines issued by the U.S. government and shown in Figure 2–2. The most common types of special and restricted diets are described here:

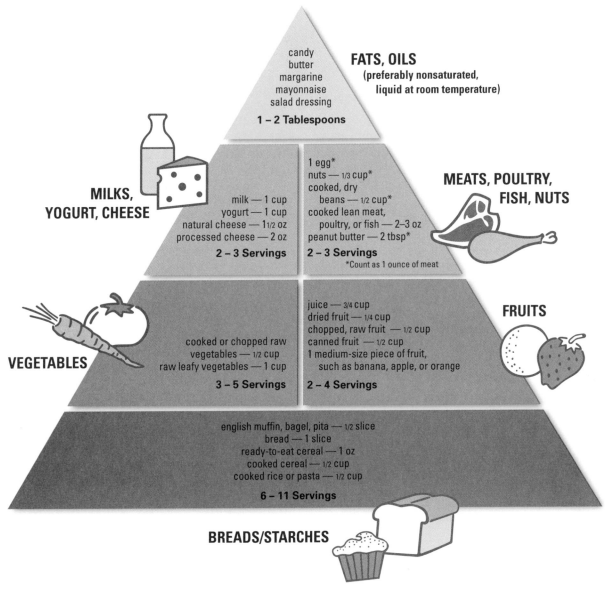

FATS, OILS
(preferably nonsaturated, liquid at room temperature)

candy
butter
margarine
mayonnaise
salad dressing
**1 – 2 Tablespoons**

MILKS,
YOGURT, CHEESE

milk — 1 cup
yogurt — 1 cup
natural cheese — 1½ oz
processed cheese — 2 oz
**2 – 3 Servings**

MEATS, POULTRY,
FISH, NUTS

1 egg*
nuts — ⅓ cup*
cooked, dry
   beans — ½ cup*
cooked lean meat,
   poultry, or fish — 2–3 oz
peanut butter — 2 tbsp*
**2 – 3 Servings**
*Count as 1 ounce of meat

VEGETABLES

cooked or chopped raw
vegetables — ½ cup
raw leafy vegetables — 1 cup
**3 – 5 Servings**

FRUITS

juice — ¾ cup
dried fruit — ¼ cup
chopped, raw fruit — ½ cup
canned fruit — ½ cup
1 medium-size piece of fruit,
   such as banana, apple, or orange
**2 – 4 Servings**

english muffin, bagel, pita — ½ slice
bread — 1 slice
ready-to-eat cereal — 1 oz
cooked cereal — ½ cup
cooked rice or pasta — ½ cup
**6 – 11 Servings**

BREADS/STARCHES

### ■ *Figure* 2–2
Nutrition pyramid.

## NPO—Nothing by Mouth

Many patients are NPO (nothing by mouth) for surgery or for diagnostic testing to prevent aspiration during procedures.

## Liquid Diet

After surgery or tests for which the patient has been NPO, he may receive clear liquids because they are easy to digest. Also, surgical patients who may be nauseated by anesthesia and pain medications tolerate clear liquids best. The clear liquid diet is missing many nutrients, but it does provide fluids.

Clear liquids include anything that you can see through, such as tea, 7-Up, apple juice, Sprite, ginger ale, Popsicles, Jell-o, sherbet, and broth. Orange juice and coffee, two of the most common drinks, should be avoided in nauseated patients because they are acidic and likely to induce vomiting. As nausea improves, the patient can be advanced to full liquids, which includes milk, ice cream, fruit juices, and cooked cereals.

## Soft Diet

A soft diet is commonly prescribed for stroke patients, patients without teeth, and patients who have had throat surgery—in short, for anyone who has trouble chewing or swallowing. Stroke patients have trouble chewing and swallowing because of paralysis. After throat surgery, patients may have problems swallowing because of pain. To make a soft diet, regular foods from the food pyramid can be put into a food processor and pureed. Patients at home may opt to buy strained baby food from the grocery store.

## Low-Fat Diet

A low-fat diet may be recommended for patients with cardiovascular disease, hypertension, or gallbladder disease. In cardiovascular disease, low-fat diets are recommended to decrease high cholesterol levels. Low-fat diets are also used to control gallbladder spasm with gallbladder disease, since fat in the intestines prompts the gallbladder to release bile to digest the fat. If the gallbladder ducts are obstructed by stones or other pathology, gallbladder spasms can be very painful and cause what is commonly called a gallbladder "attack."

## Low-Sodium Diet

Patients with cardiovascular disease are commonly put on low-sodium diets to reduce fluid retention, because anywhere sodium goes water always follows. Cardiac patients commonly retain fluids, so limited amounts of sodium are allowed in the diet to promote excretion of extra fluids. Sometimes cardiac patients are also placed on fluid restrictions.

## Low-Protein Diet

Low-protein diets are common among patients with liver and kidney failure. The liver normally metabolizes protein breakdown products, such as nitrogenous ammonia. Without conversion of ammonia to urea for excretion by the kidneys, ammonia levels build in the blood. Ammonia crosses the blood brain barrier and results in encephalopathy (malfunction of the brain), in which the patient will have symptoms such as disorientation, decreased levels of consciousness, and sensory deficits.

In renal failure, low-protein diets are also common because the kidneys are unable to excrete urea. Although the liver is functioning and produces urea, the kidneys can no longer excrete urea. Thus, levels of blood urea nitrogen (BUN) increase, urea crosses the blood brain barrier, and encephalopathy results.

## Low-Sugar Diet

Diabetic patients are unable to break down sugar (glucose) for use by any cells of the body. That means diabetics can eat very little candy, cake, pie, or other foods that contain high concentrations of sugar. Diabetes is treated by controlling the total amount of calories along with the portions of protein, fat, and carbohydrates in all food taken into the body.

Food intake must be regulated in conjunction with the quantity of insulin given, as well as the amount of daily exercise activities. Diabetics must learn to eat balanced meals and snacks that contain healthy foods low in sugar and cholesterol. Food exchange lists are based on the food pyramid as shown in Figure 2–2. They are used to show what counts as a serving of meat, fruit, milk, vegetables, or fat. For a sample daily menu, the patient may be told to eat:

- 1 fruit, 2 breads, 1 milk, and 1 teaspoon fat for breakfast
- 2 oz meat, 3 breads, 1 teaspoon fat, 1 vegetable, and 1 fruit for lunch
- 3 oz meat, 2 breads, 2 teaspoons fat, 2 vegetables for supper
- A snack of 1 milk, 1 bread and 1 teaspoon fat

## WEIGHT REDUCTION DIET

Weight reduction diets control calories while still providing all the nutrients essential for health. Healthy weight reduction diets use food exchange lists in a manner very similar to diabetic diets, balancing fruits, breads, vegetables, meats, and fats consumed during each meal. Weight reduction diets should not go below 1200 calories a day because it is nearly impossible to obtain the essential nutrients needed each day in less than 1200 calories.

Food is fuel for the body. Every activity requires fuel to produce energy. To lose weight, the patient must expend more calories than are consumed. Loss of one pound in a week will require the patient to eat 3500 calories less than needed for all activities of the body during that week.

Exercise is an important aspect of any weight reduction plan. The patient will increase the amount of energy used by burning more calories when exercising, thus improving weight loss. Added benefits besides weight loss include improved muscle tone and overall stamina. A health goal is to gradually build up to walking a minimum of 30 minutes a day, at least 4 days a week.

## HIGH-FIBER DIET

High-fiber diets are typically recommended to promote healthy bowel functioning and normal bowel movements. High-fiber foods include whole grain or bran breads and cereals, or food with skins or seeds.

## LOW-RESIDUE DIET

Patients with inflammatory bowel disease such as colitis, enteritis, or Crohn's disease commonly cannot tolerate foods high in fiber. These patients are placed on low-residue diets. Residue refers to the indigestible substances left in the gastroin-

testinal tract after digestion and absorption has occurred. With inflammation of the bowel, fibrous foods can be irritating and cause pain.

## BLAND DIET

In addition, sometimes patients with gastrointestinal or bowel problems may be placed on bland diets, which are chemically and mechanically nonstimulating. Thus, these diets include bland and soft foods.

## TUBE FEEDING

If the patient can digest food but cannot chew or swallow, he may receive food through a tube threaded into his stomach. This is called a tube feeding. The tube may be passed from the nose to the stomach (nasogastric or NG tube), or it may be surgically inserted through the abdominal wall and into the stomach (gastric tube or G tube).

A liquid food formula that contains all nutrients needed to maintain health is infused down the tube directly to the patient's stomach, bypassing the throat to avoid aspiration. The patient may have a continuous feeding, with a machine continually pumping formula at a specific hourly rate, or the patient may receive bolus feedings, in which a specific amount of formula is given all at one time. The patient typically receives a bolus at breakfast, lunch, dinner, and bedtime.

The type or brand of tube feeding, the amount to be infused in milliliters per hour, or the amount to be given in a bolus will appear in the Kardex under diet. Also, go to the patient's room or the kitchen and look at the cans of formula. Record the amount of protein, fat, and carbohydrate in each can. There are many types of food formulas designed to meet patients' special dietary needs. For example, special tube feeding formulas have been manufactured to contain reduced protein or partially digested protein for patients who have renal failure or liver failure.

## PRIORITY NUTRITION ASSESSMENTS

Patients who are confused, paralyzed, or who have decreased levels of consciousness, regardless of pathology, will need assistance and monitoring to maintain a diet successfully. These patients have trouble putting food to their mouths, chewing food, or swallowing food. If a patient cannot chew or swallow, he may choke and aspirate food into his lungs. For example, a patient who has had a stroke may be paralyzed on one side of his mouth and throat and may have decreased levels of consciousness.

Also, perform a careful assessment for a patient who has had his throat numbed because he will be temporarily unable to swallow. For example, following a bronchoscopy or endoscopy procedure, the gag reflex is temporarily paralyzed to facilitate passage of the tube into the lungs, stomach, or small intestine. Never feed someone after such a procedure until you check for a gag reflex and make sure it has returned. Also, as you consider the patient's diagnosis and procedures he has undergone, always consider the effect on the patient's ability to move his arms and place food into his own mouth as well as his ability to swallow and chew.

The patient's appetite and amount of food consumed is usually listed as a specific percentage of food eaten off a tray, such as 50% of breakfast, 25% of lunch, or 100% of supper. The amount of food consumed is generally found in the nurses' notes or on the nursing flow sheets. Flow sheets are a special form of nurses' notes used to record routine observations such as diet. In addition, any record of problems with nausea, vomiting, or diarrhea will be found in the nurses' notes.

Many patients have problems with fluid balance and need to have their fluid intake monitored to track the milliliters of fluid taken in during the shift. Fluid intake for each shift is added together to compute the fluid intake for 24 hours. Fluid intake and output will be recorded on the nursing flow sheets. Of course, fluid intake should approximately equal fluid output in a healthy state. If the patient is overhydrated and retaining fluids, she may exhibit edema. In that case, intake has exceeded output. In contrast, if the patient is dehydrated, she has lost fluids, and output has exceeded intake.

## 19. Intravenous Fluids

Fluids may also be given intravenously to replace fluids and electrolytes or to feed patients when gastrointestinal pathology prevents adequate absorption of water or nutrients. IV lines are also used to administer drugs. A small tube or catheter is inserted directly into a vein, leading from the vein to a bag of fluids. The solution flows out of the bag, through the tube, and into the vein. Nurses may regulate flow rates for IV lines manually by opening or closing a small clamp on the tubing. In many cases, the flow is controlled by an electric pump.

The type and rate of fluid for administration will be found on the Kardex. A special IV therapy record is also kept to document the entire course of IV solutions the patient has received. This record is similar to the medication record. Even if you have not yet learned how to manage an IV, it is important to note on your database that the patient has an IV line because this is the first step in relating this treatment to underlying pathology. The presence of an IV means that the patient cannot take fluids, electrolytes, nutrients, or medications orally; otherwise, the IV line would be discontinued.

There are many types of IV fluids used, such as dextrose 5% in water ($D_5W$), lactated Ringer's (LR) solution, and normal saline (NS) solution. If you do not recognize the abbreviations used in a patient's chart, one way to find out exactly what is in the bag is to look at the bag as it hangs near the patient. Once you find out what is in the bag, you can figure out how IV therapy is related to the medical and nursing diagnoses. For example, a dehydrated patient has a fluid volume deficit; therefore she is receiving dextrose and water to replace fluids.

An IV line is a potential source of infection because a catheter is going directly into the bloodstream. Therefore, nurses look carefully at where the needle is inserted under the skin and record any signs and symptoms of inflammation, such as redness, swelling, or pain at the site. The dressing over the site must be dry and intact. All of this will be noted on the IV therapy record. The total amount of IV fluids given for the day is also recorded on the nursing flow sheets under intake for the shift.

## 20. Elimination

Nurses keep track of elimination very carefully. What goes in has to come out on a regular basis, or else the patient will develop a problem. Elimination includes urine output and bowel movements.

The amount of urine in milliliters will appear on the flow sheets. Any abnormalities in urine color, odor, and quantity will be recorded in the nurse's shift assessment notes, along with pain on elimination or incontinence (loss of control over the bladder with involuntary urination).

Knowing the patient's urine output is very important. For example, patients who retain fluids have a decreased urine output that could cause or worsen problems of heart failure. Decreased urine output could also indicate renal failure. As you study the pathophysiology of disease, you will recognize how fluid volume deficits and excesses are manifestations of diseases that need to be carefully tracked. Something must be done to treat the patient if the urine output is too high or too low.

Many patients have a special tube to drain urine called a urinary catheter. The tube is usually held in place in the bladder with a balloon. In male patients, it may be held in place externally with a condom-like attachment. The tube leads to a drainage bag. Any patient who has a catheter has an elimination problem, or the tube would not be needed. You need to consider why the catheter is needed as it relates to the medical and nursing diagnoses. For example, a catheter may be needed in almost anyone with surgery of the genitourinary system to watch for bleeding in the urine and to keep track of output.

Bowel movements are also very important, because any patient who is immobilized for any reason may be prone to constipation due to decreased peristalsis. Therefore bowel movements are monitored and recorded on the flow sheets, and any abnormality is documented in the nurse's shift assessment notes. Check the flow sheet to determine when the patient last had a bowel movement, and check the nurses' notes to see about problems with constipation, diarrhea, flatus, emesis, or involuntary bowel movements.

Constipation can lead to abdominal discomfort and even impaction, where the stool creates a blockage and obstructs the bowel. If the bowel is not functioning, the patient may have problems with belching (eructation) or emesis. If gas and solid wastes cannot pass downward and out

the rectum, they will come out the other end of the gastrointestinal tract as evidenced by belching and emesis.

Postoperatively, patients typically have a decline in bowel functioning because they have been without regular meals. This decline is also due to the decrease in peristalsis that results from immobility and the adverse effects of anesthesia and narcotic pain medications. A healthy sign is the passing of flatus (gas) from the anus. Even though patients have not yet had a bowel movement, a bowel movement may be impending.

## ▄ 21. Activity

The Kardex will list the patient's activity orders. It is crucial to know what the patient can and cannot do regarding activities to keep her safe from injuries. Carefully assess the patient's ability to walk. Note the use of assistive devices such as canes, walkers, or prostheses. The patients may be ordered to bedrest, chair, bathroom privileges (commonly abbreviated as BRP), up as tolerated, and so on at the physician's discretion. Patients who are confused or have a decreased level of consciousness may need restraints or all side rails up on the bed.

In orthopedic patients, knowing the percentage of weight bearing on the injured bone is essential to prevent falls or further injury to the bone. Typically, weight bearing is described as a percentage, such as 25% on the right knee or 50% on the left hip, or toe-touch only. Abbreviations may be used for terms such as no weight bearing (NWB) or weight bearing as tolerated (WBAT).

A major concern with activity is that the patient does not fall. Preventing patient falls is a primary safety issue. Each patient has a fall risk assessment done routinely. This fall assessment is required by the JCAHO, and is a very specific standard of care. Examples of patients who are at high risk for falls include those with decreased levels of consciousness, those with sensory deficits, those receiving pain medications, and those receiving antihypertensive drugs. Review your patient's fall assessment profile, and update it to the best of your knowledge based on the data collected on the patient. If the risk for falls is great, restraints may be used for safety.

Sleeping is a very important activity. The nurses' notes will indicate whether or not the patient had any problems sleeping. Sleep is an important restorative function and promotes physical healing and cognitive function. Sleep deprivation has many negative consequences including irritability and increased sensitivity to pain.

 ## ROUTINE PHYSICAL ASSESSMENT

In inpatient or outpatient settings, routine head-to-toe physical assessment information is gathered at the beginning of the shift or on entry into the outpatient setting. You need to find the most recent physical assessment data available for the patient. Most agencies use a standardized assessment form that contains a checklist with some space for comments. Nurses expand on problem areas in the nurses' notes. When a system to be assessed is within acceptable limits, the nurse may only need to document by writing *within normal limits* (WNL) or *within designated limits* (WDL). Not writing about normal findings saves much time, and is called charting by exception. Documentation is explained in more detail in Chapter 7.

Nurses are required to perform at least one full assessment per shift and check any abnormalities in the assessment much more frequently. As you complete your database patient profile, always record the latest physical assessment data by checking the most recent physical assessment information. The following head-to-toe assessment serves as a review of important information to note on the patient profile database.

### 22. Vital Signs

Vital signs include blood pressure (BP), temperature (T), pulse (P), and respirations (R). These data provide "vital" information about the key organ systems of the body. The cardiovascular system is assessed with blood pressure and pulse, whereas the lungs are assessed with respirations. Immune functioning, specifically infection, is assessed with body temperature. The patient's most recent vital signs may be located on a temperature clipboard because they are often collected by

ancillary personnel who may not write directly on the flow sheets.

### 23. Height and Weight

Height and weight give an indication of the patient's basic nutritional status. This is found in the nursing admission assessment information.

 ## REVIEW OF SYSTEMS

In a review of systems, which is the major portion of the physical assessment, each system of the body is carefully assessed using the techniques of inspection, palpation, percussion, and auscultation. Even if you have not yet developed these assessment skills or are currently learning them, this information is vital to developing basic nursing diagnoses. Pay close attention to what has been recorded in the most recent nursing notes and nursing assessments.

### 24. Neurological and Mental Status

The functioning of the brain is assessed by determining the level of consciousness (LOC), and whether the patient is alert and oriented to person, place, and time of day or whether he is confused or disoriented. The patient's speech should be clear and appropriate. Motor status is assessed by the patient's ability to move both arms and both legs and to feel sensation, such as pressure and pain, in all limbs. The patient's pupils must be equal, round, and reactive to light and accommodation (abbreviated as PERRLA). In addition, the patient should have no deficits in the senses of hearing, vision, taste, or smell. Deficits in any of these areas place the person at high risk for injury as a primary diagnosis. Other nursing diagnoses may include **Self-care Deficit**, **Disturbed Sensory Perception**, **Impaired Verbal Communication**, **Acute or Chronic Confusion**, and **Impaired Memory**.

### 25. Musculoskeletal System

Musculoskeletal problems will be classified under the nursing diagnoses **Activity Intolerance** and **Impaired Physical Mobility**. Deficits in bones, muscles, and joints usually occupy one of the following categories:

- **Fracture**—any type of break or crack in a bone
- **Contracture**—tightening and shrinking of the muscles from paralysis or fibrosis
- **Arthritis**—inflammation of a joint
- **Spinal curvature**—deformed twisting of the bones of the spine

Circulation is another important aspect of the musculoskeletal database. A circulation check is an assessment of blood flow to the extremities. Most important, circulation checks include the distal pulses such as the pedal and tibial pulses in the feet and the radial pulse in the wrist. During the assessment, the nurse observes for pallor, warmth or coolness of the skin, the patient's sense of touch on the injured limb, the amount of edema or swelling in the limb, and amount of pain reported.

Pulse is the most important source of data about circulation to the limbs. If a pulse is not palpable, a Doppler machine is used to amplify the sound of the pulse in the artery. Lack of a pulse in a limb is a medical emergency. It means that there is no blood circulating to the limb; the tissues will die without oxygen. If the situation is not immediately rectified, it may result in the need to amputate the limb.

When bones are broken, the patient may need a cast, splint, brace, collar, or other device to immobilize muscles, tendons, or bones. Anyone in a cast needs circulation checks as described previously. Sometimes edema causes a cast to become too tight, cutting off circulation in the limb. The cast will need to be removed to restore circulation, or else there will be risk of tissue death and the need for amputation of the affected extremity.

Therapeutic treatment devices are often required to improve circulation in the limbs. Circulation decreases when the patient is immobilized. With immobility, blood stagnates in the limbs, raising the risk of serious complications such as thrombus formation, thrombophlebitis, and embolism. A thrombus is a blood clot in the leg veins that irritates and inflames the vessel (thrombophlebitis). If the thrombus breaks off and floats freely in the bloodstream, it is called an embolus and can subsequently lodge in a blood vessel in the lung (pulmonary embolism). The reason for treating patients with antiembolic stockings, mechanical plexi pulses, or sequential compression devices is to improve venous circulation and blood return to the heart, thereby preventing thrombus formation.

## ■ 26. Cardiovascular System

The basic assessment of the heart includes listening to heart sounds and determining if the sounds are normal or abnormal, determining if the heart is beating regularly or irregularly, and assessing for chest pain. Heart sounds and rate are assessed at the apical area of the heart, but a thorough assessment includes listening in the aortic, pulmonic, tricuspid, and mitral areas as well. Abnormal heart sounds and rates appear under the nursing diagnosis **Decreased Cardiac Output**. An indication of congestive heart failure, where the heart is no longer pumping fluids effectively, is engorgement of the neck veins. Engorged neck veins are referred to as jugular venous distention (JVD).

Assessment of the peripheral vascular system includes assessing all pulses, the same as during the musculoskeletal assessment. Pulses in the limbs are especially important to check because doing so helps you assess the heart's ability to pump blood to the extremities. If the pulses are not palpable, using the Doppler device to hear them is the appropriate procedure to ensure adequate circulation in the limb.

The color of the nail beds and capillary refill in the nails are indications of circulation as well. The nail beds should be pink. After depressing a nail bed, which evacuates the blood and turns the nail white, the pink color should return within 3 seconds after you stop depressing the nail bed. This is called capillary refill time.

Edema indicates that a patient is retaining fluid because the failing heart is not able to efficiently pump the fluids, so some of the fluid filters into the surrounding tissues. Pitting edema means that when the examiner compresses the edematous area with his thumb over a bone, a dent remains in the tissue for a period of time, which indicates excessive fluid in the tissues.

## ▰ 27. Respiratory System

The depth, rate, rhythm, and use of accessory muscles should be carefully observed and the breath sounds auscultated for abnormalities. Breath sounds are normally clear, without crackles (rales) or wheezes. Cyanosis, or a blue discoloration of the skin or nail beds, indicates a lack of oxygen. A cough may be characterized as productive (producing sputum) or nonproductive (without sputum). When sputum is present, the color and amount will also be recorded.

Oxygen therapy is commonly given to treat insufficient oxygenation, and the type of therapy will be listed on the Kardex or record. Oxygen is commonly given via a nasal cannula (in which small tubes extend into the patient's nostrils), a face mask, or a tracheotomy collar. Because oxygen is quite drying to mucous membranes, it often is humidified. Note the flow rate if the patient has oxygen running.

A pulse oximeter is commonly used to evaluate oxygen saturation of hemoglobin. Record the percentage of oxygen saturation. Also, note whether the patient has a history of smoking. Nursing diagnoses commonly used for problems in this area include **Impaired Gas Exchange** and **Ineffective Airway Clearance**.

## ▰ 28. Gastrointestinal System

Bowel sounds must be present in all four quadrants of the patient's abdomen. They represent peristalsis, defined as the movement of materials through the gastrointestinal (GI) tract. Bowel sounds in all four quadrants indicate a functional GI tract. Absent or decreased bowel sounds may produce a firm and distended abdomen from solid wastes and gas accumulating in the abdomen. The patient may report abdominal pain and tenderness. Decreased peristalsis may result in nausea and vomiting.

A common treatment for patients with little or no peristalsis is a nasogastric tube. This tube is inserted into the stomach and attached to suction to remove solids, fluids, and gases until bowel functioning can be returned to normal. Drainage is carefully measured as part of the patient's output. The color of the output is also carefully described. For example: brown, black, or coffee ground drainage may be caused by old dried blood, whereas green indicates bile in the drainage.

Some patients may have an ostomy, which is a surgically made opening across the abdominal wall. The intestine is cut and sewn onto the opening in the abdomen. If the ostomy involves the colon, the opening is called a colostomy. If it involves the ileum portion of the intestine, it is called an ileostomy. A plastic bag is glued to the abdomen to catch the wastes that would normally be evacuated from the rectum. This surgical procedure is usually done to treat cancer of the bowel, when the cancerous portion of the bowel is removed. The color, consistency, and amount of drainage from the ostomy will be recorded in the nurses' notes. In addition, the amount of drainage will be recorded on the flow sheet and tallied in the total patient output for the shift.

## ▰ 29. Skin and Wounds

The skin assessment includes inspection for color and turgor, along with inspection for rashes, bruises, pressure ulcers, surgical wounds, and any other type of wound (such as bullet holes or knife wounds). Describe the size and location of the wound and whether the edges are approximated. Also note if the wound is held together with sutures, staples, Steri-strips, or other material. A rash may indicate an allergy to a drug or other substance. Bruising may indicate problems with slowed blood clotting. Any type of wound or ulcer must be carefully assessed for infection, and notations must be made in the nurses' notes regarding the progress (or lack of progress) with healing the wound.

When wounds are covered with a dressing, the nurse will note whether the dressing is clean, dry, and intact. Drainage is carefully described for color and quantity. Sometimes a drain is placed inside the wound to facilitate removal of fluids and promote healing. The drainage tube is connected to a small fluid collection container such as a Jackson-Pratt bulb or a Hemovac. Jackson-Pratt and Hemovac are different brand names for drainage collection devices.

Skin assessments also involve checking for possible skin breakdown and development of pressure ulcers (also know as decubitus ulcers or pressure sores). The Braden scale or a similar rating form is used to predict the risk that a patient will develop a pressure ulcer; it is routinely completed on each patient. Factors predisposing a patient to pressure ulcers include:

- Inability to feel pain
- Skin that remains moist from perspiration or urine
- Lack of activity, such as when confined to bed
- Lack of mobility and ability to change body positions
- Poor nutrition
- The need to be moved up in bed, which can increase the risk of injury from friction and shear

The JCAHO has specified that all patients be assessed for their risk of impaired skin integrity. Therefore, you need to find the form used for assessing skin breakdown on your assigned patient and update it as needed based on the most current data you have collected on the patient.

### 30. Eyes, Ears, Nose, and Throat

The nurse will record data about the patient's eyes, ears, nose, and throat, primarily related to the inspection for signs and symptoms of infection. Infections of these structures are common and bothersome. The signs and symptoms of infection include pain in the form of aching, soreness, or itching, along with redness, drainage, and edema.

## PSYCHOSOCIAL AND CULTURAL ASSESSMENT

Without talking with the patient, only a small amount of data may be collected regarding a patient's psycho-social-cultural background. The face sheet contains general information on religious preference, marital status, insurance information, and occupation. Psychosocial and cultural assessments will be further discussed in Chapter 6, which involves mapping of psychosocial problems.

### 31. Religious Preference

Religion is an important aspect of culture. Many patients practice a religion, such as Judaism, Bud-

dhism, Islam, or Christianity. Of course, there are many variations within and between religious groups. Religious beliefs may influence a patient's view of sickness and the types of treatments that he finds acceptable. Religious beliefs also commonly influence dietary practices. And religious beliefs commonly involve rituals associated with death and dying.

### 32. Marital Status

Marital status gives one indication of the structure of the patient's family that can be easily obtained the night before clinical. A major function of a healthy family is to be supportive of each other. Spouses need to be included in the care plan, because they commonly participate in the care of the patient in the health-care agency and in the home. Determining marital status is one element of the assessment of the social support system.

### 33. Insurance

The type of insurance the patient carries directly influences what will and will not be paid for regarding medications, treatments, surgeries, or other procedures. In addition, insurance may or may not cover extended care or rehabilitation services. Knowing what will be covered by insurance is crucial to development of the care plan. A key question to think about is whether any community services are available to help the patient obtain services for which she cannot afford to pay on her own.

### 34. Occupation

Occupation gives an indication of the patient's social status, income, and educational level. During your clinical day with the patient, you will need to assess further regarding when or if the patient will be able to return to work. By finding out the patient's occupation, you can begin thinking about how the person's ability to work will be affected by her health problems.

### 35. Emotional State

The emotional assessment is very important, so check the nurses' notes for notations about the patient's mood. Mood is a reflection of emotions, such as anxiety, hopelessness, powerlessness, and ineffective coping. If you are permitted to meet your patient the day before clinical and introduce yourself, you can make a direct observation of the patient's mood for your records. Does the patient appear happy? Sad? Quiet? Nervous? Write down your impressions on the database.

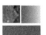 **OBTAINING STANDARDIZED FORMS**

### 36. Additional Information

Before leaving the clinical agency the night before clinical (or at the beginning of the clinical day), gather all the standardized forms that pertain to your patient. These are printed materials that are used by the health-care agency on patients that have the same diagnosis as your patient.

### STANDARDIZED SKIN ASSESSMENT

The purpose of the standardized skin assessment is to prevent pressure ulcers by estimating the patient's risk of developing them. The risk level is based on mental status, continence, mobility, activity, and nutrition. Those at highest risk have decreased levels of consciousness; incontinence; immobility; bedridden status; and inadequate intake of nutrients. You should know what your patient's risk is for development of an ulcer and develop a plan for preventing this problem. Use the standardized form to estimate your patient's risk for pressure ulcer formation. You will include how to prevent pressure ulcers in the plan of care.

### STANDARDIZED FALLS-RISK ASSESSMENT

The purpose of the standardized falls-risk assessment is to prevent injury. The risk to patients is based partly on mental status, with those patients who are confused and disoriented at highest risk. Another risk involves illness-related debilitation, causing patients to be light-headed when standing, especially during the first 24 hours postoperatively. Patients with orthostatic hypotension are at risk as well, as are patients with visual impairments, mobility problems, and an unsteady gait. In addition, many patients take

medications, such as sedatives and narcotics, that increase their risk for falling. You should use the standardized falls-risk assessment form to estimate your patient's risk of falling. Preventive measures related to falls should be incorporated into the nursing plan of care.

### STANDARDIZED NURSING CARE PLANS

Many agencies have developed standardized nursing care plans for many common medical diagnoses. The care plans include the typical nursing diagnoses, expected patient outcomes, and nursing interventions.

### CLINICAL PATHWAYS

Clinical pathways (also known as critical pathways) are standard care plans that integrate all disciplines involved in a patient's care. This type of care planning has come about because of managed health care. The purpose of a clinical pathway is to coordinate services and decrease costs. Physicians, nurses, physical therapists, nutritionists, and other professionals jointly specify typical problems, interventions, and expected outcomes on a day-by-day basis for a specific disease or condition.

Pathways are in the process of development in many agencies, and you may or may not have pathways to follow. If pathways are being used, make sure you know exactly where your patient is on the pathway for the day you will be providing care. Analyze your patient's progress on the pathway to determine whether she is on time, behind the estimated schedule, or ahead of schedule. If she is ahead or behind, try to determine the reason for the variation.

### PATIENT EDUCATION MATERIALS

Patient education is an important aspect of nursing care. Many agencies have developed patient education materials; others use printed booklets. Audiovisual aids may also be available. Take these materials home with you and study them. Integrate them into your plan of care. Be prepared to review educational materials with your patient as appropriate during the clinical day of care.

## COMMUNICATING WITH NURSING STAFF

Try to get as much patient information as possible on your own, and keep a list of questions about any information you cannot find on your patient. Then discuss that list in detail with your clinical faculty. Many students hesitate to bother nursing staff or other personnel in the agency when they are gathering data to prepare a plan of care. But most busy nurses do not mind answering a few thoughtful questions; after all, they were students too at one time. Keep in mind, however, that it is your responsibility to gather the relevant data. It is a learning experience for you to be searching out the information on your own, with clinical supervision from the faculty.

Once you have gathered information from the written records, find the nurse who is responsible for caring for your patient on the day of the assignment. Somewhere in the agency is an assignment sheet that shows all the patient assignments. When you find your patient's nurse, introduce yourself as a student nurse assigned to that patient on the following day. Then ask a very simple open-ended question, such as, "Is there anything special I should know about this patient?" Chances are you will get some good information that may not be written down anywhere. You may even be able to ask one or two more "quick" questions if the nurse has time. Many nurses are glad to have students' help in caring for their patients, and most do not mind answering brief questions if time allows. If the nurse is very busy, she may not have time to talk with you. If so, do not take it personally. The nurses do not know you, and they are busy. Save your remaining questions for your clinical faculty.

## CHAPTER SUMMARY

Gathering data is a time-consuming process, at least initially. The good news is that it gets easier each time you do it because you become more familiar with where to find the information. And the only way you can develop a comprehensive plan of care is to make sure you have complete, accurate assessment data. Sound clinical judgments result from excellent assessments and data analysis.

Your patient profile database comes mainly from your review of patient records. Record keeping in health-care agencies is generally excellent, thanks to standards established by the JCAHO and the American Nurses Association. In fact, data about patients is required to be accessible, recorded, and communicated.

The initial patient profile database is focused on pathophysiology and treatments, and it has psychological, social, and cultural components. This chapter describes the essential components of the basic patient profile database, the purpose of each component, and where the information is likely to be found in the medical records. The patient's current health problems and history of problems need to be identified, along with information from a head-to-toe physical assessment. In addition, treatments, medications, intravenous therapy, laboratory values, and diagnostic tests need to be identified and related to the patient's health problems. Diet and activity are also important aspects of treatment that need to be identified. In addition, the effects of the health alterations on growth and development, emotional state, and the type of discomforts typically caused by the patient's health problem are very important aspects of the initial assessment.

## LEARNING ACTIVITIES

1. Go on a field trip with your clinical group and your clinical faculty to a hospital or outpatient setting. Locate and review the following records: patient charts and information contained in them, such as the face sheet, consent forms, laboratory data, and diagnostic test data; medication records; IV records; the Kardex; nursing flow sheets; nursing assessments; and nurses' notes. Find out where to get the most recent information for each item. For example, perhaps the most recent laboratory data is kept in a special place in the front of the chart. This may vary from agency to agency and even from unit to unit within the agency.

2. After completing exercise 1, work alone or with another student to complete a patient profile database using Figure 2–1 on a real patient.

3. As you gather patient data, keep a list of abbreviations that were confusing and need clarification. Usually, each unit has its own set of abbreviations in addition to the standard abbreviations found in most textbooks. Hundreds of abbreviations are used inconsistently and create confusion. For example, DAT may mean diet as tolerated, and BKA may mean below the knee amputation. Write down anything that confuses you, and ask your faculty for clarification. Share your list with others in the clinical group.

4. Find out where the list of patient assignments is posted and track down the staff nurse responsible for your patient. Be assertive and ask how the patient is doing today. Go into the patient's room and introduce yourself. Ask the patient how he is doing and if you can get him anything. Stay no longer than 5 minutes. If the patient asks for something you cannot do or provide, you will need to tell the nurse. The point of this exercise is to determine what you can assess about your patient's emotional state in just five brief minutes by listening to him and watching his nonverbal behavior.

## REFERENCES

1. Standards of Nursing Clinical Practice, ed 2. American Nurses Publishing, American Nurses Foundation/ American Nurses Association, Washington, D.C., 1998.
2. Erickson, EH: Childhood and Society. Norton, New York, 1963.
3. Schuster, PM: Communication: The Key to the Therapeutic Relationship. FA Davis, Philadelphia, 2000.
4. Tannen, D: You Just Don't Understand: Women and Men in Conversation. Ballantine, New York, 1990.
5. Malarkey, LM, and McMorrow, ME: Nurses Manual of Laboratory Tests and Diagnostic Procedures. WB Saunders, Philadelphia, 2000.
6. Malarkey, LM, and McMorrow, ME: Op cit.

# Chapter 3

## Concept Mapping:
### Grouping Clinical Data in a Meaningful Manner

## OBJECTIVES

1. Identify the American Nurses Association nursing standard of care related to organizing patient data.
2. Identify primary medical diagnoses.
3. Review patient profile data to determine general health problems.
4. Categorize patient profile data under health problems resulting from the patient's response to the health problem.
5. List primary assessments associated with the medical diagnosis.
6. Label nursing diagnoses.
7. Specify relationships between nursing diagnoses.

*A*fter gathering assessment of data, the next step in care planning is to develop the concept map. When you finish, the map will contain the primary medical and nursing diagnoses for your patient and all the supporting data categorized neatly under the appropriate nursing diagnoses. In addition, relationships between diagnoses will be identified on the map.

In this chapter, the focus is on the American Nurses Association (ANA) standard of practice 2, which states that nursing diagnoses are to be derived from the health data.[1] Concept maps promote critical analysis of health data in a way that increases the probability of formulating nursing diagnoses accurately. Students are sometimes too quick to put diagnostic labels on patients without data to support the diagnosis, resulting in diagnostic errors. Concept maps help students to correctly organize data, and thus improve the accuracy of the nursing diagnoses.

You will follow three basic steps to develop a concept map. These steps are based on meaningful learning theory and assimilation theory.[2,3] The first step is to map out propositions. The second step is to arrange data in hierarchical order. The third step is to make meaningful associations between segments of the map. In this chapter, these theoretical steps will be defined with concrete examples for application to nursing care plans.

Students are sometimes confused by the word theory. However, theories are very important because they explain phenomena. Meaningful learning theory and assimilation theory explain how you can increase your critical-thinking abilities by mapping concepts. Concept mapping is a useful method for helping nursing students to clinically reason and formulate clinical judgments during analysis and organization of patient profile data. Students demonstrate critical thinking when logically organizing data in a concept map. Critical-thinking skills are used during the process of developing maps.

This chapter is intended to give you practice in developing concept maps for three different patient scenarios: a patient with diabetes, a surgical patient with a knee replacement, and a surgical patient with a mastectomy. Patient profile data will be provided for each scenario. You will be guided step by step in completing a concept map in the first scenario. Scenarios 2 and 3 are included at the end-of-chapter exercises for additional practice in developing concept maps.

## Scenario 1

### Database for Patient with Diabetes

Figure 3–1 contains data that was collected by a student nurse from a patient's records. The patient was hospitalized with newly diagnosed diabetes. The patient profile database is sketchy, but it contains all the information this student collected. Let's assume the student has not had much experience in collecting data, and this is her first patient assignment. Carefully review the information in Figure 3–1 to obtain some general ideas about the patient's problems that will be used for Step 1 of concept mapping. As you review the database, ignore the blank questions for now. The first step is to formulate initial impressions of the clinical patient profile data.

### STEP 1: Develop a Basic Skeleton Diagram

In Step 1 of concept mapping, you will map the framework of propositions. You must propose or state what you believe to be your patient's key problems based on the data you collected. The key problems are also known as the concepts. The framework is the diagram of the key problems, the first step in creating the concept map. Do this step *before* you start to look up information in your reference materials. Start by centering the medical diagnosis on a blank page:

> **Newly Diagnosed Diabetes**

Next, think about the big problems the medical diagnosis has created for this patient, based on the assessment data. He has problems with diet and nutrition; he has elimination problems; he is anxious; he hasn't yet learned enough about how to manage his care at home; and he has an ongoing medical problem of hypertension. Put these problems around the medical diagnosis, like spokes on a wagon wheel:

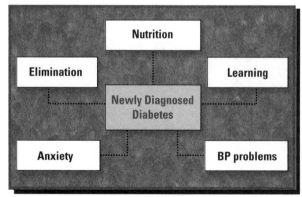

The next task is to look up information on medical diagnoses, medications, and treatments. The aim of looking up this information is to develop a general understanding of what is wrong with the patient and what is being done by the physician to correct the patient's problems. Let's assume this is the first patient you have ever been assigned to care for. You are in your first clinical course, and

# PATIENT PROFILE DATABASE

## ADMISSION INFORMATION

Student Name: *Nancy Nurse*

| ❶ Date of Care: | ❷ Patient Initials: | ❸ Age: | ❸ Growth and Development: | ❹ Sex: | ❺ Admission Date: |
|---|---|---|---|---|---|
| *3/23* | *ET* | (face sheet) *80* | *Ego integrity vs. despair* | (face sheet) *M* | (face sheet) *3/21* |

**❻ Reason for Hospitalization** (face sheet):

*Diabetes*

**❼ Medical Diagnoses:** (present diagnoses, past diagnoses; physician's History and Physical notes in chart; nursing intake assessment and Kardex)

**❽ Surgical Procedures** (consent forms and Kardex):

*New onset diabetes (defined above}*
*History of hypertension*

---

**Medical Dx:**

**Etiology:**

**Signs and symptoms:**

**Complications:**

**Usual treatment goals:**

**Nursing implications:**

---

**Medical Dx:**

**Etiology:**

**Signs and symptoms:**

**Complications:**

**Usual treatment goals:**

**Nursing implications:**

---

## ❾ ADVANCE DIRECTIVES (NURSE'S ADMISSION ASSESSMENTS):

Living will: ☐ yes ☐ no    Power of attorney: ☐ yes ☐ no    Do not resuscitate (DNR) order (Kardex): ☐ yes ☐ no

## ❿ LABORATORY DATA

| Test | Norms | On admission | Current value | Test | Norms | On admission | Current value |
|---|---|---|---|---|---|---|---|
| White blood cells | | | | Potassium | | | |
| Differential | | | | Blood Glucose | | *450* | *120* |
| Hemoglobin | | | | Glycohemoglobin | | *12%* | |
| Hematocrit | | | | Cholesterol | | *240* | |
| Platelets | | | | Low-density lipoproteins | | | |
| Prothrombin time | | | | Urine analysis | | *3+ sugar, no ketones, no protein, no WBCs, clear yellow* | |
| International normalized ratio | | | | | | | |
| Activated partial thromboplastin time | | | | Other abnormal | | | |

*What are the normal values for each test? How is each test used to diagnose and monitor diabetes?*

---

■ *Figure* 3–1

Scenario 1. Patient newly diagnosed with diabetes: Patient profile database.

*(Continued)*

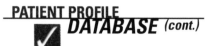
## ⑪ DIAGNOSTIC TESTS

| Chest x-ray: | EKG: | Other abnormal reports: |
|---|---|---|
| Other: | Other: | Other: |

## ⑫ MEDICATIONS   *List medications and times of administration (medication administration record and check the drawer in the carts for spelling):*

| Medication/Time of Administration | Medication/Time of Administration | Medication/Time of Administration |
|---|---|---|
| *Humulin N 35 U q.* A.M., *7:30* A.M. | *Valsartan 80 mg q.* A.M., *9* A.M. | *Acetaminophen 650 mg, q4h, p.r.n.* |

**Humulin**        *Generic and brand name?:*                    *What is it used for?:*
*Adverse reactions/side effects to monitor for?:*
*What must be assessed before giving the drug?:*
*Onset, duration, peak action?:*

**Valsartan**        *Generic and brand name?:*                    *What is it used for?:*
*Adverse reactions/side effects to monitor for?:*
*What must be assessed before giving the drug?:*
*Onset, duration, peak action?:*

**Acetaminophen**        *Generic and brand name?:*                    *What is it used for?:*
*Adverse reactions/side effects to monitor for?:*
*What must be assessed before giving the drug?:*
*Onset, duration, peak action?:*

## ALLERGIES / PAIN

| ⑬ **Allergies** (medication administration records): **None known** | ⑭ **When was the last pain medication given?** (medication administration record): **None given** |
|---|---|
| ⑭ **Where is the pain?** (nurse's notes): | ⑭ **How much pain is the patient in on a scale from 0 – 10?** (nurse's notes, flow sheet): |

## TREATMENTS

| ⑮ **Treatments** (Kardex): *Accu-check q.i.d., ac & hs* *VS q4h* | ⑯ **Support services** (Kardex): *Dietary* | ⑰ **Consultations** (Kardex): *Diabetes educator* |
|---|---|---|

*What is Accu-check?:*
*Why are VS needed q4h?:*
*What will the dietitian do for the patient? Be specific:*
*What does the diabetes educator teach the patient? Be specific:*

## ⑱ DIET / FLUIDS

| Type of Diet (Kardex): *1800 ADA* | Restrictions (Kardex): *No sugar added* | Gag reflex intact: ☒ yes ☐ no | Appetite: *Good* | Breakfast *100* % | Lunch *100* % | Supper *100* % |
|---|---|---|---|---|---|---|

*What type of diet is this?:*
*What does ADA stand for?:*
*What type of foods are included in this diet and what foods should be avoided?:*

■■ ***Figure* 3–1** *(continued)*

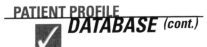

## 18  DIET / FLUIDS (cont.)

| | |
|---|---|
| Fluid intake:<br>24 hours<br>(flow sheet) | 2200 |
| Tube feedings:<br>type and rate<br>(Kardex) | N/A |

*Circle Those Problems That Apply:*

- **Problems: swallowing, chewing, dentures** (nurse's notes)
- **Needs assistance with feeding** (nurse's notes)
- **Nausea or vomiting** (nurse's notes)
- **Overhydrated or dehydrated** (evaluate total intake and output on flow sheet)
- **Belching**
- **Other:** *history of polyphagia*

> What is polyphagia?:
>
> Why is the patient's intake greater than output?:
>
> Why is intake always compared to output?:

## 19  INTRAVENOUS FLUIDS (IV therapy record)

| Type and rate:<br><br>N/A | IV dressing dry, no edema, redness of site:<br><br>☐ yes  ☐ no | Other: |
|---|---|---|

## 20  ELIMINATION (flow sheet)

| Last bowel movement: | 24-hour urine output:<br>1800 | Foley/condom catheter:<br>☐ yes  ☐ no |
|---|---|---|

*Circle Those Problems That Apply:*

- **Bowel:**    constipation    diarrhea    flatus    incontinence    belching
- **Urinary:**    hesitancy    frequency    burning    incontinence    odor
- **Other:** *history of polyuria*

> What is polyuria?:
>
> How does polyuria relate to diabetes?:
>
> Why is the urine output only 1800 when intake is 2200?:

## 21  ACTIVITY (Kardex, flow sheet)

| Ability to walk (gait): | Type of activity orders:<br>OOB/chair | Use of assistive devices: cane,<br>walker, crutches, prosthesis: | Falls-risk assessment rating:<br>at RISK (see chart below) |
|---|---|---|---|
| No. of side rails<br>required (flow sheet):   2 | Restraints (flow sheet):<br>☐ yes  ☒ no | Weakness:<br>☒ yes  ☐ no | Trouble sleeping (nurse's notes):<br>☐ yes  ☒ no |

> What does OOB/chair mean?:
>
> Why isn't the patient up ad lib?:
>
> Why would diabetes cause weakness?:

## PHYSICAL ASSESSMENT DATA

| 22  BP (flow sheet):<br>138/92 | 22  TPR (flow sheet):<br>98.4-77-18 | 23  Height: _5'10"_    Weight: _174 lb_    (nursing intake assessments) |
|---|---|---|

> What are the normal values for BP?:
>
> What are the normal values for TPR?:
>
> What is normal height and weight for a male 5'10"?:

**Figure 3–1** *(continued)*

**24 NEUROLOGICAL/MENTAL STATUS:** _WNL_

| LOC: alert and oriented to person, place, time (A&O x 3) confused, etc. *alert and oriented to person, place, time (A&O x 3)* | Speech: clear, appropriate/inappropriate |
|---|---|
| Motor: ROM x 4 extremities | Sensation: 4 extremities | Pupils: PERRLA | Sensory deficits for vision/hearing/taste/smell *glasses* |

**25 MUSCULOSKELETAL SYSTEM:** _WNL_

| Bones, joints, muscles (fractures, contractures, arthritis, spinal curvatures, etc.): | Extremity circulation checks (pulses, temperature, sensation, edema): |
|---|---|
| Ted hose/plexi pulses/compression devices: type: | Casts, splint, collar, brace: |

**26 CARDIOVASCULAR SYSTEM:** _WNL_

| Pulses (radial, pedal) (to touch or with Doppler): | Capillary refill (<3 s): ☐ yes ☐ no | Edema, pitting vs. nonpitting: |
|---|---|---|
| Neck vein (distention): | Sounds: $S_1$, $S_2$, regular, irregular: | Any chest pain: |

**27 RESPIRATORY SYSTEM:** _WNL_

| Depth, rate, rhythm: | Use of accessory muscles: | Cyanosis: | Sputum: color, amount: | Cough: productive, nonproductive: | Breath sounds: clear, rales, wheezes: |
|---|---|---|---|---|---|
| Use of oxygen: nasal cannula, mask, trach collar: | Flow rate of oxygen: | Oxygen humidification: ☐ yes ☐ no | Pulse oximeter: _____ % oxygen saturation | Smoking: ☐ yes ☐ no | |

**28 GASTROINTESTINAL SYSTEM:** _WNL_

| Abdominal pain, tenderness, guarding; distention, soft, firm: | Bowel sounds x 4 quadrants: | NG tube: describe drainage: |
|---|---|---|
| Ostomy: describe stoma site and stools: | Other: | |

**29 SKIN AND WOUNDS:** _WNL_

| Color, turgor: | Rash, bruises: | Describe wounds (size, location): | Edges approximated: ☐ yes ☐ no | Type of wound drains: |
|---|---|---|---|---|
| Characteristics of drainage: | Dressings (clean, dry, intact): | Sutures, staples, steri-strips, other: | Risk for decubitus ulcer assessment rating: | Other: |

**30 EYES, EARS, NOSE, THROAT (EENT):** _WNL_

| Eyes: redness, drainage, edema, ptosis | Ears: drainage | Nose: redness, drainage, edema | Throat: sore |
|---|---|---|---|

### PSYCHOSOCIAL AND CULTURAL ASSESSMENT:

| 31 Religious preference (face sheet): *Catholic* | 32 Marital status (face sheet): *Widower* | 33 Health-care benefits and insurance (face sheet): *Blue Cross/Blue Shield* | 34 Occupation (face sheet): *Retired* | 35 Emotional state (nurse's notes): *Anxious about giving insulin and following diet* |
|---|---|---|---|---|

Additional information to obtain from clinical units the night before clinical specific to your patient's diagnosis:

| Standardized falls-risk assessment: ☐ yes ☐ no | Pressure ulcer assessment: ☐ yes ☐ no | Standardized skin assessment: ☐ yes ☐ no | Standardized nursing care plans: ☐ yes ☐ no | Clinical pathways: ☐ yes ☐ no | Patient education materials: ☐ yes ☐ no |
|---|---|---|---|---|---|

■ *Figure* **3–1** *(continued)*

you are learning assessment and fundamentals of nursing, including medication administration.

It is now appropriate to attempt to answer some questions about the information in Figure 3–1. You will need to use course textbooks and software to look up information. Reference materials may include a medical dictionary, a manual of laboratory and diagnostic procedures, a book on nutrition therapy, a drug handbook or pharmacology book, a standardized care plan book, a fundamentals textbook, and medical-surgical textbook. In addition, you may use software programs and Internet sites that decrease the amount of time it takes to look up materials, such as computerized drug guides[4] or computerized nursing care plans.[5] There is also an Internet site, *www.ask.com*, to learn about any topic. Go to the site, ask any question, and you will get an answer! For example, go to the site and ask for patient education for diabetes and you will find all kinds of information in an instant.

### Looking Up Information

For this patient, you will need to look up information about drugs, laboratory and diagnostic tests, diet, and medical diagnoses.

#### Drugs

Start by looking up drugs. There are only three for this patient. You may be thinking, "Why start with drugs?" Medication administration is one of the most dangerous things nurses do, and it is a primary focus of fundamentals courses. Therefore, before you use up all your energy looking up everything else, invest some time when your mind is fresh reading and taking some notes on the drugs. Think about what the patient needs to know about taking his drugs properly when he gets home.

#### Laboratory and Diagnostic Tests

Next, read about the laboratory and diagnostic tests in a laboratory and diagnostic procedures manual. Medication administration is often based on laboratory values. There is a direct relationship between the laboratory values and the patient's medication. You must identify those relationships. Make sure you know the most up-to-date laboratory values before you administer drugs. Also, identify what the patient needs to know about the diagnostic tests that have been ordered.

#### Diet

Third, get information on the patient's prescribed diet. How is the diet related to the medical diagnosis? What does the patient need to know about his diet? What is a sample menu for the patient? If you have a nutritional therapy book, at least one chapter will be devoted to diabetes. If you do not have a nutrition book, this would be a good topic on which to try the *www.ask.com* Web site. Ask for information about diabetic diets.

#### Medical Diagnoses

Last but certainly not least in importance is to find information about the patient's medical diagnoses. Your fundamentals text may not offer much help here, because many fundamentals books contain little disease-specific information. The aim of a fundamentals text is to teach foundational skills essential for providing care of basic human needs. Fundamentals courses typically do not cover specific aspects of medical-surgical nursing care. Therefore, you may find a medical dictionary helpful to briefly define the disease, symptoms, etiology, complications, treatments, prognosis, and nursing implications.

You'll find the most detailed information about diseases in a medical-surgical nursing text. In fact, it is a good investment to buy a medical-surgical text ahead of time so you can use the book as a reference in your fundamentals course. You may find certain Web sites helpful as well, such as those shown in Box 3–1.

Other helpful references include standardized care plan guidelines and clinical pathways. These may be obtained from the health-care agency or from standardized care planning manuals.[6] These standardized care plans include patient goals, patient outcomes, nursing interventions, and rationales. Clinical pathways also integrate the services of other health professionals in attaining patient goals. These are general guidelines, not specific to a particular patient. The concept map care plan that you develop will be specific to your patient on the day you care for him.

| **Box 3–1** | *WEB SITES: GATHERING INFORMATION* |
|---|---|

| | |
|---|---|
| American Heart Association | www.americanheart.org |
| Arthritis Foundation | www.arthritis.org |
| National Cancer Institute | www.cancernet.nic.nih.gov |
| American Diabetes Association | www.diabetes.org |
| Immunization Action Coalition | www.immunize.org |
| American Lung Association | www.lungusa.org |
| Mental Health InfoSource | www.mhsource.org |
| Nephron Information Center | www.nephron.com |
| Neurosciences on the Internet | www.neuroguide.com |
| National Organization for Rare Disorders | www.rarediseases.org |

As you review standardized plans and pathways, you must sort through all the possible nursing diagnoses, goals, objectives and interventions; then you must determine what is appropriate for the day you are assigned to care for the patient. This has been called individualizing the plan of care. This is difficult at first, but with practice and experience, you will get better at it. Selecting goals, objectives, and interventions for the day of care will be the focus of Chapter 4. In summary, a very important point to remember as you review information from standardized plans is that you must determine what is most relevant to the patient at the point in time you are assigned to care for him.

### Preventing Falls and Skin Breakdown

The next step in building a concept map for your diabetic patient is to analyze his risk for falls and skin breakdown. As you know, preventing falls and skin breakdown is fundamental to competent nursing care. In fact, the Joint Commission on Accreditation of Healthcare Organizations (JCAHO) requires that all patients be evaluated for falls and skin breakdown, so each agency you work in will have assessment forms for this task. Samples of assessment forms with data from the case study in this chapter are shown in Figures 3–2 and 3–3. These have been filled out based on patient profile data and also based on what is known about patients with diabetes. Thus, the specifics of the data collected and the general information for a patient with diabetes is used to complete the assessments. You must rate your patient for falls and skin breakdown based on the most current information you obtained on the patient.

When assessing the patient's risk of falling, as shown in Figure 3–2, consider that the patient is over age 60, he's weak, he has had problems with urinary frequency, and he's taking an antihypertensive.[7] By looking up information, you may conclude that his weakness is from inadequate nutrition and dehydration. Urinary frequency is associated with the polyuria, the antihypertensive drug may contribute to orthostatic hypotension, and decreased muscle tone and strength may be associated with aging. Therefore, this patient is at risk for a fall.

Next, assess the patient's risk for development of a pressure ulcer. As explained in Chapter 2, each patient is assessed for potential problems in development of skin breakdown. This breakdown is termed a pressure ulcer or decubitus ulcer.

Figure 3–3 shows the Braden Scale for Predicting Pressure Sore Risk.[8] To assess a patient's risk, you will score the patient on each of the six subscales and total the points. The maximum score is 23, which indicates little or no risk. A score between 10 and 16 indicates a risk of pressure ulcer. And a score of 9 or less indicates a high risk of pressure ulcer.

How would you rate the diabetic patient in this scenario? Based on data from the patient's profile, the patient does not have any sensory impairments (4 points); he is probably rarely moist (4 points); probably walks occasionally

# RISK FOR FALLS ASSESSMENT

DIRECTIONS: Place an "x" in front of elements that apply to your patient. Based on the assessment, check whatever applies to the patient. A patient for whom you place four or more "x" marks is at risk for falling

## MEDICATIONS

___ Diuretics or diuretic effects
_X_ Hypotensive or CNS suppressants drugs
___ Postoperative/admitted for operation (e.g., narcotic, sedative, psychotropic, hypnotic, tranquilizer, antihypertensive, antidepressant)
___ Medication that increases GI motility

## GENERAL DATA

_X_ Age over 60
___ History of falls before admission
___ Postoperative/admitted for operation
___ Smoker

## AMBULATORY DEVICES USED

___ Cane
___ Crutches
___ Walker
___ Wheelchair
___ Geriatric (geri) chair
___ Braces

## PHYSICAL CONDITION

___ Dizziness/imbalance
___ Unsteady gait
___ Diseases/other problems effecting weight-bearing joints
_X_ Weakness
___ Paresis
___ Seizure disorder
___ Impairment of vision
___ Impairment of hearing
___ Diarrhea
_X_ Urinary frequency

## MENTAL STATUS

___ Confusion/disorientation
___ Impaired memory or judgment
___ Inability to understand or follow directions

■ *Figure* 3–2

Risk for falls assessment. (From Brians LK, et al: The development of the RISK tool for fall prevention. Rehabilitation Nursing 1991:16(2):67, with permission.)

# BRADEN SCALE >>> FOR PREDICTING PRESSURE SORE RISK

| Patient's Name: | Evaluator's Name: | Date of Assessment: |
|---|---|---|

| | **1** | **2** | **3** | **4** |
|---|---|---|---|---|
| **SENSORY PERCEPTION** Ability to respond meaningfully to pressure-related discomfort | **Completely limited:** Unresponsive (does not moan, flinch, or grasp) to painful stimuli, due to diminished level of consciousness or sedation, OR limited ability to feel pain over most of the body surface. | **Very Limited:** Responds only to painful stimuli. Cannot communicate discomfort except by moaning or restlessness, OR has a sensory impairment which limits the ability to feel pain or discomfort over 1/2 of the body. | **Slightly Limited:** Responds to verbal commands but cannot always communicate discomfort or need to be turned, OR has a sensory impairment which limits ability to feel pain or discomfort in 1 or 2 extremities. | **No Impairment:** Responds to verbal commands. Has no sensory deficit which would limit ability to feel or voice pain or discomfort. |
| **MOISTURE** Degree to which skin is exposed to moisture | **Constantly Moist:** Skin is kept moist almost constantly by perspiration, urine, etc. Dampness is detected every time patient is moved or turned. | **Moist:** Skin is often but not always moist. Linen must be changed at least once a shift. | **Occasionally Moist:** Skin is occasionally moist, requiring an extra linen change approximately once a day. | **No Impairment:** Responds to verbal commands. Has no sensory deficit which would limit ability to feel or voice pain or discomfort. |
| **ACTIVITY** Degree of physical activity | **Bedfast:** Confined to bed. | **Chairfast:** Ability to walk severely limited or nonexistent. Cannot bear own weight and/or must be assisted into chair or wheelchair. | **Walks Occasionally:** Walks occasionally during day but for very short distances, with or without assistance. Spends majority of each shift in bed or chair. | **Walks Frequently:** Walks outside the room at least twice a day and inside room at least once every 2 hours during walking hours. |
| **MOBILITY** Ability to change and control body position | **Completely Immobile:** Does not make even slight changes in body or extremity position without assistance. | **Very Limited:** Makes occasional slight changes in body or extremity position but unable to make frequent or significant changes independently. | **Slightly Limited:** Makes frequent though slight changes in body or extremity position independently. | **No Limitations:** Makes major and frequent changes in position without assistance. |
| **NUTRITION** Usual food intake pattern | **Very Poor:** Never eats a complete meal. Rarely eats more than 1/3 of any food offered. Eats 2 servings or less of protein (meat or dairy products) per day. Takes fluids poorly. Does not take a liquid dietary supplement, OR is NPO and/or maintained on clear liquids or IVs for more than 5 days. | **Probably Inadequate:** Rarely eats a complete meal and generally eats only about 1/2 of any food offered. Protein intake includes 3 servings of meat or dairy products per day. Occasionally will take a dietary supplement, OR receives less than optimum amount of liquid diet or tube feeding. | **Adequate:** Eats over half of meals. Eats a total of 4 servings of protein (meat, dairy products) each day. Occasionally will refuse a meal, but will usually take a supplement if offered, OR is on a tube feeding or TPN regimen, which probably meets most of nutritional needs. | **Excellent:** Eats most of every meal. Never refuses a meal. Usually eats a total of 4 or more servings of meat and dairy products. Occasionally eats between meals. Does not require supplementation. |
| **FRICTION AND SHEAR** | **Problem:** Requires moderate to maximum assistance in moving. Complete lifting without sliding against sheets is impossible. Frequently slides down in bed or chair, requiring frequent repositioning with maximum assistance. Spasticity, contractures, or agitation leads to almost constant friction. | **Potential Problem:** Moves feebly or requires minimum assistance. During a move skin probably slides to some extent against the sheets, chair, restraints, or other devices. Maintains relatively good position in chair or bed most of the time but occasionally slides down. | **No Apparent Problem:** Moves in bed and in chair independently and has sufficient muscle strength to lift up completely during move. Maintains good position in bed or chair at all times. | |

■ *Figure* 3–3

Braden scale for pressure ulcer assessment. (From Braden, B, and Bergstrom, N: In Bryant, RA (ed): Acute and Chronic Wounds: Nursing Management. Mosby, St. Louis, 1992.)

(3 points); probably has slightly limited mobility from being only out of bed and in a chair (OOB/chair) (3 points); has excellent nutrition (4 points); and has a potential problem with friction and shear (2 points). He has 20 of 23 points based on the evidence provided in the patient profile database. Thus, he has a low risk for developing a pressure ulcer.

At this point, you have completed the patent profile database and looked up basic information about the disease and its treatment. It is now time to categorize all the data you have gathered under the basic problems you identified on your map. All the pieces of data must be organized into a hierarchical and comprehensive pattern.

## STEP 2: Analyze and Categorize Data

According to educational theory, concept maps are hierarchical graphical organizers. A hierarchy is a series of consecutive classes or groups. For example, one hierarchy in biology is the classification of living things into kingdom, phylum, class, order, family, genus, and species. Subconcepts are organized in a pattern under major concepts, to facilitate understanding of relationships and to organize information. The graph of the hierarchy is a picture or map of the organized relationships between concepts and subconcepts.

In concept map care planning, the subconcepts are the specific pieces of data that were collected about the patient and that support the major problems you identified on the spokes of the wheel surrounding the medical diagnosis. The subconcepts that must be classified are the clinical signs and symptoms the patient displayed, treatments, medications, and medical history data collected. You must sift through the data once more and categorize it.

Keep in mind that a concept map is based on actual problems. Consequently, you should categorize only real patient data. This is one reason why it is important for you to look up information on the patient's disease, drugs, treatments, and so on before categorizing the data; that way, you have general knowledge of the main treatments for the primary medical diagnosis.

The problems that extend out from the central medical diagnosis will become nursing

diagnoses based on the definitions and classifications of the North American Nursing Diagnosis Association (NANDA).[9] Categorize all the data you have *before* assigning any diagnostic labels. After categorizing all the data, then you can attach the diagnostic label.

Start by reviewing the physical assessment data, and try categorizing physical assessment data in appropriate boxes. If an item belongs in more than one box, put it in two or more places. If you do not know where an item goes, place it in a corner of the map. At this stage of development your map would look like this:

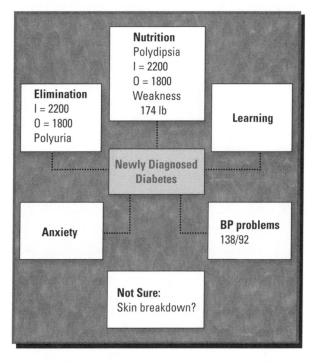

Now try to add remaining pieces of data items into your boxes. For example, add information about drugs (humulin N, valsartan, acetaminophen), lab tests (serum glucose 450 down to 120, glycosylated hemoglobin = 12%, cholesterol = 240, urine 3+ sugar), treatments (Accucheck, VS q.i.d.), diet (1800 American Diabetes Association [ADA], no added sugar), activity (OOB/chair, risk of falls), and psychosocial-cultural data (**Anxiety** diagnosis, injections and diet, widower). Now your map might look something like the box on p. 56.

You must be able to explain why you put each item in the box you selected based on what you read about the pathophysiology of

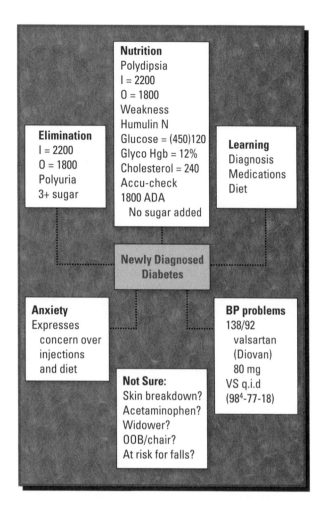

widower, and skin breakdown. This means you have not collected enough data to make decisions about those items, and you need to do more assessment when you meet with the patient the next day. For example, you'll need to find out whether the acetaminophen was prophylactic and never used. Did the patient have pain somewhere? Was he running a temperature?

Since he is a widower, what type of social support does he have? The answer to this question could have major implications if the patient has no one at home to help him accomplish the self-care tasks the patient cannot accomplish on his own. He may need nursing home placement or home health care.

And what about the skin breakdown? He doesn't have any specific problems noted in the data, but from your reading you may have noted that diabetics have trouble with circulation and sensation in their legs and feet, making them prone to skin breakdown. What's more, their wounds heal slowly. The patient needs to be taught foot care and methods to prevent skin breakdown.

### Adding Assessments for Primary Medical Diagnoses

Now that you have pretty much all of your patient data arranged on your concept map, you should add key assessments to the central box that contains the medical diagnosis. These are important assessments, relating specifically to the medical diagnoses, that you will focus on while you are with the patient. The results of these assessments will tell you whether the patient is making progress toward a healthier state in which his diabetes is under control.

In a patient with diabetes, the key assessments are to watch for hypoglycemia or hyperglycemia and to assess blood glucose levels. Hypoglycemia typically causes weakness, dizziness, sluggishness, hunger, irritability, sweating, paleness, a rapid heart rate, tremors, headache, and changes in mental functioning, such as confusion. The classic signs of hyperglycemia and ketosis are polydipsia (excessive thirst), polyuria (excessive urination), and polyphagia (excessive appe-

the patient's disease, monitoring of the disease, and treatment of the disease.

A number of items are listed off to the corner that didn't seem to fit in any of your original boxes. If you look at these items as a group, they suggest that the patient is not as mobile as he should be, and he has a risk of falling. This realization warrants adding another box to your map to address the patient's mobility problem. The symptom of weakness also goes along with this problem of mobility.

> **Mobility**
> Risk of falls
> OOB/chair
> Weakness

Suppose you are still not sure about the remaining items in the box: acetaminophen, tite). The potential for hypoglycemia in the hospital setting is high until food intake, exercise, and the amount of insulin the patient receives are in careful balance.

In short, the most important problem to watch for in this patient would be an insulin reaction. When giving the patient his insulin, make sure you know his blood glucose level, and make sure he is going to eat if you are giving a premeal dose. Always monitor vital signs. The center of the map would look like this:

> **Newly Diagnosed Diabetes**
> Signs and symptoms of hypoglycemia and hyperglycemia; monitor blood glucose, food intake, VS

These additions are integrated into the final map that appears on page 60.

### STEP 3: Label Diagnoses—Analyze Relationships between Problems

#### Labeling Nursing Diagnoses

Remember to attach nursing diagnoses labels to problems *after* carefully considering all of the data. Many students have a tendency to select nursing diagnoses too quickly, without first looking at and organizing all the data. The net result of making quick decisions about diagnoses is that the diagnoses are often wrong. Therefore, take time to look at the data before you leap into the diagnoses.

Assigning correct diagnoses is essential to developing an individualized plan of care that includes appropriate goals, outcome objectives, and interventions specific to the day you are assigned to care for the patient. In other words, it will be impossible to develop an individualized plan if you have not accurately identified and prioritized the patient's specific problems. Once you have identified the problems correctly, it is relatively easy to find information on what to do to correct those problems. Developing the plan of care once the correct diagnoses are made is the subject of Chapter 4.

Nursing diagnoses are statements that describe the patient's actual or potential responses to health problems or life processes that the nurse is licensed and competent to treat.[10-15] Nursing diagnoses are focused on the patient's responses to a health problem. In contrast, medical diagnoses are focused on the health problem itself, based on the signs and symptoms related to the pathophysiology of the disease. Medical and nursing diagnoses are inextricably linked, and you—as the nurse—must recognize the linkages. The linkages between the medical and nursing diagnoses are clearly shown by the lines between the medical and nursing diagnoses on the concept map. The nursing diagnoses flow outward from the primary medical diagnosis like spokes on a wheel. You will continue to grow in your knowledge of nursing diagnoses and medical diagnoses with each day of clinical experience.

For the medical diagnosis of diabetes, the resulting general problems that you identified are elimination, nutrition, learning, anxiety, blood pressure problems, and immobility. These are the problems that you believe to be the patient's actual responses to the health problem of diabetes. In concept map care planning, the focus is on actual problems, not potential problems. The concept map is based strictly on real data. There are many potential problems in any patient care situation, but the concept map is focused on actual problems.

In the NANDA system, the nursing diagnoses have been placed into a framework that groups them in categories and makes them easier to locate. Nursing diagnoses have been arranged according to Maslow's hierarchy of self-actualization needs (see Appendix A), which include:

- Self-esteem
- Love and belonging
- Safety and security
- Physiological needs[16]

They have also been organized according to Gordon's Functional Health Patterns (see Appendix B), which include:

- Health-perception–health-management pattern
- Nutritional-metabolic pattern
- Elimination pattern
- Activity-exercise pattern
- Sleep-rest pattern
- Cognitive-perceptual pattern

- Self-perception–self-concept pattern
- Role-relationship pattern
- Sexuality-reproductive pattern
- Coping-stress tolerance pattern
- Value-belief pattern[17]

A third popular framework is NANDA's Human Response Patterns, which include:

- Exchanging
- Communicating
- Relating
- Valuing
- Choosing
- Moving
- Perceiving
- Knowing and feeling[18]

Each nursing diagnosis you select for your map must be based on an accurate assessment of the patient's problems. Use the appendixes at the back of the book to locate possible diagnoses for the problems you identified. Review Maslow's Hierarchy (Appendix A), Gordon's Functional Health Patterns (Appendix B), and NANDA's classification system (Appendix C). Appendix C includes definitions for diagnoses that are not self-explanatory.

### Elimination

The data we have to support the problem is the patient's polyuria, which is a classic symptom of hyperglycemia. In addition, the patient is spilling glucose into his urine, also a classic sign of hyperglycemia. Also, the patient's output is currently less than his input, which is likely to be a compensatory response by the body to the dehydrated state caused by polyuria. A review of the list of nursing diagnoses indicates the diagnosis of **Impaired Urinary Elimination** is probably correct. To confirm the diagnosis, look up its definition, which says, "the state in which the individual experiences a disturbance in urine elimination."[19] This fits well with the data you have collected.

### Nutrition

A patient with diabetes definitely has nutritional problems. This patient is on the 1800-calorie diabetic diet with no added sugar and is receiving insulin to regulate his blood glucose.

Accu-check is being used regularly to monitor his blood glucose level, and his glycosylated hemoglobin is elevated. In addition, the patient's cholesterol is elevated, a problem that should be controlled to decrease his risk of coronary artery disease. The patient's records indicate that he had polydipsia and that currently his intake exceeds output, probably to compensate for the dehydration that occurred before he was regulated with replacement of insulin. The weakness is related to the starvation and dehydration that occurred without adequate insulin. Although the patient appears to be getting better, the diagnosis of **Imbalanced Nutrition: Less Than Body Requirements** is appropriate. It says, "the individual is experiencing an intake of nutrients insufficient to meet metabolic needs."[20]

### Learning

All newly diagnosed patients with any disease need to learn about self-care. In this case, the patient needs to learn about the disease, how to prevent complications such as through foot care, medications such as insulin, the 1800 ADA diet, and exercise. Foot care and exercise would be added to the box that addresses patient learning needs. The appropriate diagnosis is **Deficient Knowledge**. The definition says, "absence or deficiency of cognitive information related to a specific topic."[21]

### Anxiety

The patient said that he is anxious about learning to give himself injections and about following his diet. The diagnosis of **Anxiety** is defined as "a vague uneasy feeling of discomfort or dread accompanied by an autonomic response; the source is often nonspecific or unknown to the individual; a feeling of apprehension caused by anticipation of danger. It is an alerting signal that warns of impending danger and enables the individual to take measures to deal with threat."[22] At this point, the patient appears to be a little anxious, probably because he doesn't know what is involved or if he will be capable of caring for himself.

### Mobility

The patient has an increased risk of falling caused by weakness, and he is permitted to be

OOB/chair. He can be diagnosed with **Impaired Physical Mobility**, which is defined as a "limitation in independent, purposeful physical movement of the body or of one or more extremities."[23]

### Blood Pressure (BP) Problems

He is receiving a blood pressure medication and has a slightly elevated diastolic blood pressure. Diabetes affects blood vessels all over the body, and most diabetics eventually develop cardiovascular disease and peripheral vascular disease. An appropriate nursing diagnosis is **Ineffective Tissue Perfusion (peripheral),** defined as "a decrease in oxygen resulting in the failure to nourish the tissues at the capillary level."[24] The patient will need instruction on slowing down the process of peripheral vascular complications, although these complications are inevitable. Peripheral vascular complications of diabetes will affect circulation and sensation in the extremities, with skin breakdown and ulcerations as common consequences of the disease. Healing of wounds is much slower than normal if the person has diabetes. It is clear now that the skin breakdown risk that you put in a box in the corner of the map would fit well with altered tissue perfusion. Your map should now look something like this:

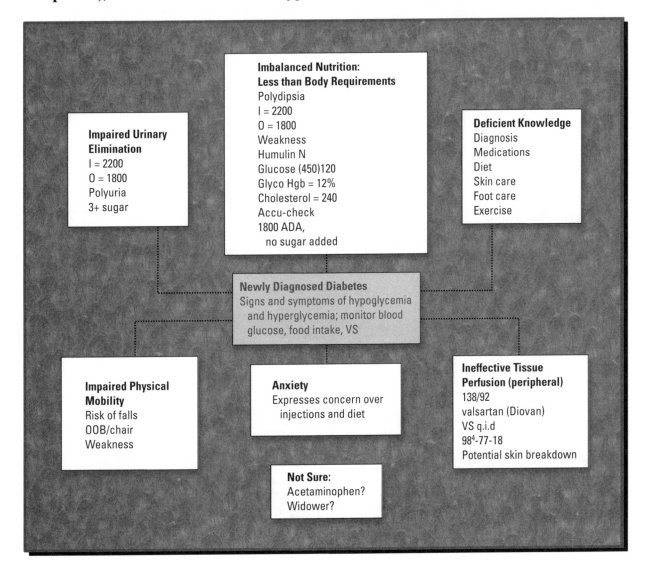

**Imbalanced Nutrition:**
**Less than Body Requirements**
Polydipsia
I = 2200
O = 1800
Weakness
Humulin N
Glucose (450)120
Glyco Hgb = 12%
Cholesterol = 240
Accu-check
1800 ADA,
 no sugar added

**Impaired Urinary Elimination**
I = 2200
O = 1800
Polyuria
3+ sugar

**Deficient Knowledge**
Diagnosis
Medications
Diet
Skin care
Foot care
Exercise

**Newly Diagnosed Diabetes**
Signs and symptoms of hypoglycemia and hyperglycemia; monitor blood glucose, food intake, VS

**Impaired Physical Mobility**
Risk of falls
OOB/chair
Weakness

**Anxiety**
Expresses concern over injections and diet

**Ineffective Tissue Perfusion (peripheral)**
138/92
valsartan (Diovan)
VS q.i.d
98⁴-77-18
Potential skin breakdown

**Not Sure:**
Acetaminophen?
Widower?

Your concept map is almost complete. You need just one more thing. Step 3 of concept mapping involves analyzing the relationships between the nursing diagnoses. The objective is to make meaningful associations between one concept on the map and other concepts on the map. The links must be accurate, meaningful, and complete. In concept map care planning, the concepts you must link are the nursing diagnoses.

You must be able to explicitly state why you believe the diagnoses are related. Your faculty will be able to look at your map and

see what was (or was not) in your mind and ask you questions about the relationships you indicated. So be prepared with good answers. Your final map should now look like Figure 3–4.

Your explanations of the primary relationships between nursing diagnoses will be based on your knowledge of the disease process, as in the following examples.

**Imbalanced Nutrition** and **Impaired Urinary Elimination**: These two concepts are always linked in any disease. What goes in and is metabolized must come out in equal

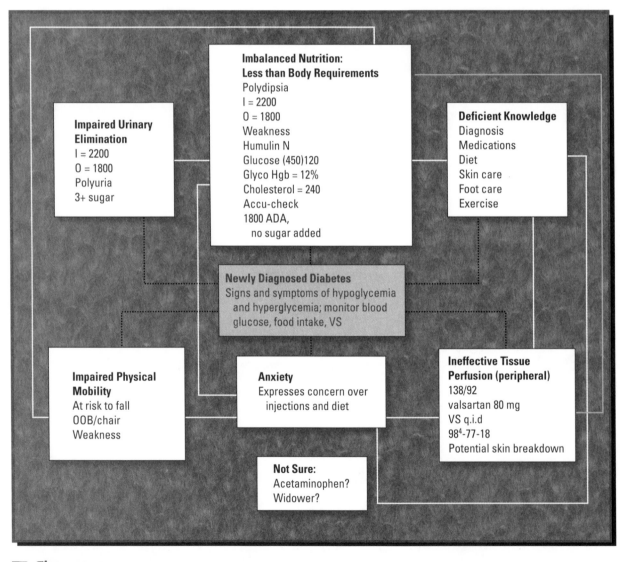

**Impaired Urinary Elimination**
I = 2200
O = 1800
Polyuria
3+ sugar

**Imbalanced Nutrition:**
**Less than Body Requirements**
Polydipsia
I = 2200
O = 1800
Weakness
Humulin N
Glucose (450)120
Glyco Hgb = 12%
Cholesterol = 240
Accu-check
1800 ADA,
    no sugar added

**Deficient Knowledge**
Diagnosis
Medications
Diet
Skin care
Foot care
Exercise

**Newly Diagnosed Diabetes**
Signs and symptoms of hypoglycemia
and hyperglycemia; monitor blood
glucose, food intake, VS

**Impaired Physical Mobility**
At risk to fall
OOB/chair
Weakness

**Anxiety**
Expresses concern over
    injections and diet

**Ineffective Tissue Perfusion (peripheral)**
138/92
valsartan 80 mg
VS q.i.d
98$^4$-77-18
Potential skin breakdown

**Not Sure:**
Acetaminophen?
Widower?

■ *Figure 3–4*

amounts or there will be a health problem. Metabolism is altered with diabetes because a lack of insulin causes blood glucose to rise and excess glucose to spill into the urine. As glucose is excreted, water is pulled out of the body by osmosis, creating an osmotic diuresis. Osmosis is the process by which a solution of higher concentration will pull water across a semipermeable membrane to equalize the concentrations on both sides of the membrane. Currently, the patient is making up for losses that created a state of dehydration by retaining fluids. Thus, at this point, the intake exceeds output.

**Imbalanced Nutrition** and **Impaired Physical Mobility**: Without adequate nutrition, the body becomes weak and debilitated, leading to impaired physical mobility.

**Imbalanced Nutrition** and **Ineffective Tissue Perfusion:** High blood glucose damages to peripheral blood vessels, which in turn leads to problems with tissue oxygenation and nerve damage, leading to hypertension, cardiovascular disease, peripheral neuropathies, nephropathies, foot ulcers, and infections.

**Ineffective Tissue Perfusion** and **Impaired Physical Mobility**: Tissue perfusion problems, treatment with an antihypertensive, and neuropathies all influence this patient's mobility, giving him an increased risk of falling and an increased risk of skin breakdown.

**Deficient Knowledge**, **Anxiety**, **Ineffective Tissue Perfusion**, and **Imbalanced Nutrition**: Anxiety is common in newly diagnosed patients, no matter which health problem is involved. Anxiety may result from self-doubts about performing self-care and making lifestyle changes. Knowledge of the disease and treatments may serve to decrease the patient's anxiety. The key things the patient must learn are primarily related to nutrition and tissue perfusion. The patient will need to learn about the disease itself, including signs and symptoms, dietary management, blood glucose checks, insulin administration, exercise, and skin and foot care.

## CHAPTER SUMMARY

**Important note:** The diagnoses on the night before clinical are primarily physiological, but should always include anticipated knowledge deficits and psychosocial-emotional problems such as anxiety if you have the assessment data to support it. The focus of the initial plan is based only on data that is recorded and perhaps a brief introduction to your patient and a brief chat with the staff nurse.

Typically, little is formally written about the psychosocial-cultural assessment unless you are in a psychiatric setting. The psychosocial-cultural assessment is much less formal than the physiological assessment in most care settings, including home care settings. You must spend time with the patient to do the psychosocial-cultural assessment; then you can add psychosocial-cultural diagnoses to the concept map on the day you care for the patient. This will be the focus of Chapter 6, "Mapping Psychosocial Problems."

The purpose of this chapter was to take you slowly through the first three steps of the concept map care planning process. After gathering clinical data, Step 1 is to map the framework of propositions by noting the major medical diagnosis and the problems that result from that medical diagnosis. In Step 2, organize the data into a hierarchy of subordinate concepts. This involves organizing abnormal physical assessment data, treatments, medications, diagnostic and lab tests, past medical problems, and emotional state under the problems listed in Step 1. An important aspect of Step 2 is the identification of key areas of assessment related to the primary medical diagnosis. Step 3 involves the final selection of nursing diagnostic labels based on the analysis of all available data. Step 3 involves the identification of meaningful associations between concepts on the map. The relationships between the nursing diagnoses are indicated with lines. The relationships you indicate must be accurate, meaningful, and complete; you should be prepared to explain why you believe a relationship exists between two connected diagnoses. In the rest of this chapter, you will find two additional scenarios that you can use to practice Steps 1, 2, and 3 of the concept mapping process.

# LEARNING ACTIVITIES

1. Patient scenarios appear in Figures 3–5 and 3–6 at the end of this section. Develop concept maps for the data presented in these figures.
2. Compare concept map diagrams with your classmates.
3. During class, explain to your classmates why you believe relationships exist between nursing diagnoses you have connected with lines in Step 3.

# PATIENT PROFILE DATABASE

## ADMISSION INFORMATION
Student Name ...... *MAB*

| **1** Date of Care: | **2** Patient Initials: | **3** Age: (face sheet) | **3** Growth and Development: | **4** Sex: (face sheet) | **5** Admission Date: (face sheet) |
|---|---|---|---|---|---|
| 12/4 | AL | 80 | *Ego integrity vs. despair* | F | 12/3 |

**6** Reason for Hospitalization (face sheet):
*Mastectomy*

**8** Surgical Procedures (consent forms and Kardex):
*Right modified radical mastectomy*

**7** Medical Diagnoses: (present diagnoses, past diagnoses; physician's History and Physical notes in chart; nursing intake assessment and Kardex)

*Invasive carcinoma in right breast*
*NIDDM*
*Hypertension*
*MI - 1994*

## 9 ADVANCE DIRECTIVES (NURSE'S ADMISSION ASSESSMENTS):

Living will: ☐ yes ☒ no     Power of attorney: ☐ yes ☒ no     Do not resuscitate (DNR) order (Kardex): ☐ yes ☐ no

## 10 LABORATORY DATA

| Test | Norms | On admission | Current value | Test | Norms | On admission | Current value |
|---|---|---|---|---|---|---|---|
| White blood cells | | 5.6 | 4.8 | Potassium | | 2.8 | 2.8 |
| Differential | | | | Blood Glucose | | 230 | 235 |
| Hemoglobin | | 11.2 | 11 | Glycohemoglobin | | | |
| Hematocrit | | 33.2 | 33.1 | Cholesterol | | | |
| Platelets | | 259,000 | | Low-density lipoproteins | | | |
| Prothrombin time | | | | Urine analysis | | | |
| International normalized ratio | | | | | | | |
| Activated partial thromboplastin time | | | | Other abnormal | | | |

## 11 DIAGNOSTIC TESTS

| Chest x-ray: | EKG: | Other abnormal reports: |
|---|---|---|
| Other: | Other: | Other: |

## 12 MEDICATIONS
*List medications and times of administration (medication administration record and check the drawer in the carts for spelling):*

| Medication/Time of Administration | Medication/Time of Administration | Medication/Time of Administration |
|---|---|---|
| *Heparin 5000 u 10 A.M.* | *KCL (K-Dur) 20 mEq 10 A.M.* | *Ecotrin 1 tablet PO 10 A.M.* |
| *Lasix 40 mg PO 8 A.M.* | *Zoloft 25 mg PO 10 A.M.* | *K-Dur 40 mEq x 1* |
| *Tenormin 25 mg PO 10 A.M.* | *Lanoxin 0.125 mg PO 10 A.M.* | *Darvocet N-100 1 tab, q4h, p.r.n.* |
| | | |
| | | |
| | | |

■ *Figure* **3–5**

Scenario 2. A surgical patient with a mastectomy: Patient profile database.

*(Continued)*

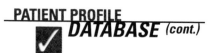

## ALLERGIES / PAIN

| | |
|---|---|
| **13** Allergies (medication administration records):  **NKA** | **14** When was the last pain medication given? (medication administration record):  **Darvocet 6 A.M., getting it sporadically** |
| **14** Where is the pain? (nurse's notes):  **surgical incision** | **14** How much pain is the patient in on a scale from 0 – 10? (nurse's notes, flow sheet):  **5, confusion makes this unreliable** |

## TREATMENTS

| | | |
|---|---|---|
| **15** Treatments (Kardex):  VS q1h x 2 then q2h x 2, then routine  I&O and record q1h x 2  Drsg – sterile gauze and surgical bra, change qA.M. | **16** Support services (Kardex):  Respiratory – Incentive spirometry q2h | **17** Consultations (Kardex): |

## 18 DIET / FLUIDS

| Type of Diet (Kardex):  1800 ADA | Restrictions (Kardex): | Gag reflex intact:  ☒ yes ☐ no | Appetite:  Eating jello and tea only | Breakfast ____ % | Lunch ____ % | Supper ____ % |
|---|---|---|---|---|---|---|

*Circle Those Problems That Apply:*

| | |
|---|---|
| Fluid intake:  24 hours  **2100**  (flow sheet) | • Problems: swallowing, chewing, ⟨dentures⟩ (nurse's notes)  ⟨• Needs assistance with feeding⟩ (nurse's notes) |
| Tube feedings:  type and rate  (Kardex) | • Nausea or vomiting (nurse's notes)  • Overhydrated or dehydrated (evaluate total intake and output on flow sheet)  • Belching        • Other: _____ |

## 19 INTRAVENOUS FLUIDS (IV therapy record)

| Type and rate:  LR with 20 mEq K per bag  @ 100 cc/hr x 2 L | IV dressing dry, no edema, redness of site:  ☐ yes ☐ no | Other:  **Pulled out IV during the night and restarted** |
|---|---|---|

## 20 ELIMINATION (flow sheet)

| Last bowel movement:  no BM since before surgery | 24-hour urine output:  1700 cc | Foley/condom catheter:  ☐ yes ☒ no |
|---|---|---|

*Circle Those Problems That Apply:*

| • Bowel: | constipation | diarrhea | flatus | incontinence | belching |
|---|---|---|---|---|---|
| • Urinary: | hesitancy | frequency | burning | incontinence | odor |
| • Other: _____ | | | | | |

## 21 ACTIVITY (Kardex, flow sheet)

| Ability to walk (gait): | Type of activity orders:  **As tolerated** | Use of assistive devices: cane, walker, crutches, prosthesis: | Falls-risk assessment rating:  **Very high – 7 confused** |
|---|---|---|---|
| No. of side rails required (flow sheet):  **4 side rails** | Restraints (flow sheet):  ☒ yes ☐ no  **vest restraints, wrist restraints** | Weakness:  ☐ yes ☐ no | Trouble sleeping (nurse's notes):  ☒ yes ☐ no |

## PHYSICAL ASSESSMENT DATA

| **22** BP (flow sheet):  137/72  152/100 | **22** TPR (flow sheet):  97 52 20  97.8 80 20 | **23**  Height: **5'5"**    Weight: **190 lb**    (nursing intake assessments) |
|---|---|---|

■ *Figure* **3–5** *(continued)*

**REVIEW OF SYSTEMS** Write WNL (within normal limits) if normal and describe abnormalities in space provided: (check nurses' notes and shift assessments for the latest information you can get)

**PATIENT PROFILE**
✓ **DATABASE** (cont.)

**② NEUROLOGICAL/MENTAL STATUS:** _____

| LOC: alert and oriented to person, place, time (A&O x 3) confused, etc. | Speech: clear, appropriate/inappropriate |
|---|---|
| *confused, oriented to person only, became confused during the evening after surgery* | *Does not know where she is* |

| Motor: ROM x 4 extremities | Sensation: 4 extremities | Pupils: PERRLA | Sensory deficits for (vision)/hearing/taste/smell |
|---|---|---|---|
| *WNL* | *WNL* | *WNL* | *glasses* |

**② MUSCULOSKELETAL SYSTEM:** _WNL_

| Bones, joints, muscles (fractures, contractures, arthritis, spinal curvatures, etc.): | Extremity circulation checks (pulses, temperature, sensation, edema): |
|---|---|
| Ted hose/plexi pulses/compression devices: type: | Casts, splint, collar, brace: |

**② CARDIOVASCULAR SYSTEM:** _WNL_

| Pulses (radial, pedal) (to touch or with Doppler): | 3+ | Capillary refill (<3 s): ☒ yes ☐ no | Edema, pitting vs. nonpitting: |
|---|---|---|---|
| Neck vein (distention): | | Sounds: $S_1$, $S_2$, regular, irregular: | Any chest pain: |

**② RESPIRATORY SYSTEM:** _WNL_

| Depth, rate, rhythm: 20 | Use of accessory muscles: | Cyanosis: | Sputum: color, amount: | Cough: productive, nonproductive: | Breath sounds: (clear), rales, wheezes: *slightly decreased in bases* |
|---|---|---|---|---|---|
| Use of oxygen: nasal cannula, mask, trach collar: | Flow rate of oxygen: | Oxygen humidification: ☐ yes ☐ no | Pulse oximeter: ____% oxygen saturation | | Smoking: ☐ yes ☐ no |

**② GASTROINTESTINAL SYSTEM:** _WNL_

| Abdominal pain, tenderness, guarding; distention, soft, firm: *soft and nondistended* | Bowel sounds x 4 quadrants: *active bowel sounds* | NG tube: describe drainage: |
|---|---|---|
| Ostomy: describe stoma site and stools: | Other: | |

**② SKIN AND WOUNDS:** _____

| Color, turgor: *skin dry and chapped, poor turgor* | Rash, bruises: | Describe wounds (size, location): *red and edematous, intact, drain sites reddened* | Edges approximated: ☒ yes ☐ no | Type of wound drains: *JP #1 25 cc, JP #2 100 cc* |
|---|---|---|---|---|
| Characteristics of drainage: *both seroanquineous* | Dressings (clean, dry, intact): *clean, dry, intact* | Sutures, staples, steri-strips, other: | Risk for decubitus ulcer assessment rating: 7 | Other: |

**③ EYES, EARS, NOSE, THROAT (EENT):** _WNL_

| Eyes: redness, drainage, edema, ptosis | Ears: drainage | Nose: redness, drainage, edema | Throat: sore |
|---|---|---|---|

**PSYCHOSOCIAL AND CULTURAL ASSESSMENT:**

| ③ Religious preference (face sheet): *Catholic* | ③ Marital status (face sheet): *Widowed* | ③ Health-care benefits and insurance (face sheet): *Medicare* | ③ Occupation (face sheet): *Housewife* | ③ Emotional state (nurse's notes): *Anxious, wants to go home, very talkative, does not respond to questions appropriately* |
|---|---|---|---|---|

**Additional information to obtain from clinical units the night before clinical specific to your patient's diagnosis:**

| Standardized falls-risk assessment: ☐ yes ☐ no | Pressure ulcer assessment: ☐ yes ☐ no | Standardized skin assessment: ☐ yes ☐ no | Standardized nursing care plans: ☐ yes ☐ no | Clinical pathways: ☐ yes ☐ no | Patient education materials: ☐ yes ☐ no |
|---|---|---|---|---|---|

■ **Figure 3–5** (continued)

# PATIENT PROFILE
## *DATABASE*

### ADMISSION INFORMATION          Student Name __BCD__

| **1** Date of Care: | **2** Patient Initials: | **3** Age: (face sheet) | **3** Growth and Development: | **4** Sex: (face sheet) | **5** Admission Date: (face sheet) |
|---|---|---|---|---|---|
| 2/5 | PUD | 55 | *Generativity vs. Stagnation* | M | 2/4 |

**6** Reason for Hospitalization (face sheet):
*Total knee arthroplasty*

**7** Medical Diagnoses:(present diagnoses, past diagnoses; physician's History and Physical notes in chart; nursing intake assessment and Kardex)

**8** Surgical Procedures(consent forms and Kardex):
*Total knee arthroplasty*

*Arthritis, chronic pain in rt knee*
*Hx hypertension*

### **9** ADVANCE DIRECTIVES (NURSE'S ADMISSION ASSESSMENTS):

Living will: ☐ yes ☒ no    Power of attorney: ☐ yes ☒ no    Do not resuscitate (DNR) order (Kardex): ☐ yes ☒ no

### **10** LABORATORY DATA

| Test | Norms | On admission | Current value | Test | Norms | On admission | Current value |
|---|---|---|---|---|---|---|---|
| White blood cells | | 4.8 | | Potassium | | | |
| Differential | | | | Blood Glucose | | | |
| Hemoglobin | | 11.5 | | Glycohemoglobin | | | |
| Hematocrit | | 35.3 | | Cholesterol | | | |
| Platelets | | 173,000 | | Low-density lipoproteins | | | |
| Prothrombin time | | 11.5 | | Urine analysis | | | |
| International normalized ratio | | | | | | | |
| Activated partial thromboplastin time | | 22.1 | | Other abnormal | | | |

### **11** DIAGNOSTIC TESTS

| Chest x-ray: | EKG: | Other abnormal reports: |
|---|---|---|
| Other: | Other: | Other: |

### **12** MEDICATIONS    List medications and times of administration (medication administration record and check the drawer in the carts for spelling):

| Medication/Time of Administration | Medication/Time of Administration | Medication/Time of Administration |
|---|---|---|
| *K-Dur 20 mEq b.i.d.* | *Lovenox 30 mg q.d.* | *Vicodin I or 2 po q3-4h p.r.n. pain* |
| *Hytrin 5 mg q.d.* | *Kefzol IV 1 gm, q.d.* | *Tigan IM q6h p.r.n. n/v* |
| *Colace 100 mg q.d.* | *Demoral 75 mg IM q3-4h p.r.n. pain* | |
| | | |
| | | |
| | | |

■ *Figure* 3–6

Scenario 3. A surgical patient with a knee replacement: Patient profile database.          *(Continued)*

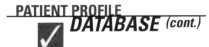

## ALLERGIES / PAIN

**13** **Allergies** (medication administration records): *sulfa, tetanus*

**14** **When was the last pain medication given?** (medication administration record): *11:20 P.M. Demoral, 4 A.M. and 8 A.M. vidocin 2*

**14** **Where is the pain?** (nurse's notes): *surgical incision*

**14** **How much pain is the patient in on a scale from 0 – 10?** (nurse's notes, flow sheet): *8, down to 2 after meds*

## TREATMENTS

**15** **Treatments** (Kardex):
*CPM q shift 3 h*
*Mini pillow under ankle*
*Plexi-pulses*
*Overhead frame and trapeze*
*Ice pack to knee*

**16** **Support services** (Kardex):
*Respiratory – IS q2h with C&DB*
*Physical therapy:*
*teaches to use walker, CPM*

**17** **Consultations** (Kardex):
*1800 ADA*

## 18 DIET / FLUIDS

| Type of Diet (Kardex): | Restrictions (Kardex): | Gag reflex intact: | Appetite: | Breakfast | Lunch | Supper |
|---|---|---|---|---|---|---|
| *Regular* | | ☒ yes ☐ no | | _75_ % | _50_ % | _75_ % |

*Circle Those Problems That Apply:*

Fluid intake:
24 hours
(flow sheet)  *1072*

Tube feedings:
type and rate
(Kardex)

- **Problems: swallowing, chewing, dentures** (nurse's notes)
- **Needs assistance with feeding** (nurse's notes)
- **Nausea or vomiting** (nurse's notes)
- **Overhydrated or dehydrated** (evaluate total intake and output on flow sheet)
- **Belching**
- **Other:** _____

## 19 INTRAVENOUS FLUIDS (IV therapy record)

Type and rate:
*autotransfusion,*
*D5W 1/2NS 1000 cc q12h*

IV dressing dry, no edema, redness of site:
☒ yes ☐ no

Other:

## 20 ELIMINATION (flow sheet)

| Last bowel movement: | 24-hour urine output: | Foley/condom catheter: |
|---|---|---|
| *2/3* | *875 cc* | ☒ yes ☐ no |

*Circle Those Problems That Apply:*

- **Bowel:** constipation    diarrhea    flatus    incontinence    belching
- **Urinary:** hesitancy    frequency    burning    incontinence    odor
- **Other:** _____

## 21 ACTIVITY (Kardex, flow sheet)

| Ability to walk (gait): | Type of activity orders: | Use of assistive devices: cane, walker, crutches, prosthesis: | Falls-risk assessment rating: |
|---|---|---|---|
| *unsteady* | *WBAT* | *walker* | *6 – is at risk* |

No. of side rails
required (flow sheet): *2*

Restraints (flow sheet):
☐ yes ☒ no

Weakness:
☒ yes ☐ no

Trouble sleeping (nurse's notes):
☐ yes ☒ no

## PHYSICAL ASSESSMENT DATA

**22** **BP** (flow sheet): *124/66*

**22** **TPR** (flow sheet): *36.3 (celcius) 72/20*

**23** Height: _5'11"_    Weight: _201 lb_    (nursing intake assessments)

■ *Figure* **3–6** *(continued)*

## REVIEW OF SYSTEMS

*Write WNL (within normal limits) if normal and describe abnormalities in space provided: (check nurses' notes and shift assessments for the latest information you can get)*

**24 NEUROLOGICAL/MENTAL STATUS:** _WNL_

| LOC: alert and oriented to person, place, time (A&O x 3) confused, etc. | | | Speech: clear, appropriate/inappropriate |
|---|---|---|---|
| | | _WNL_ | _WNL_ |

| Motor: ROM x 4 extremities | Sensation: 4 extremities | Pupils: PERRLA | Sensory deficits for ⟨vision⟩/hearing/taste/smell |
|---|---|---|---|
| _Decreased in rt knee_ | _WNL_ | _WNL_ | _glasses_ |

**25 MUSCULOSKELETAL SYSTEM:** _____

| Bones, joints, muscles (fractures, contractures, arthritis, spinal curvatures, etc.): _Arthritis rt knee and arthroplasty_ | Extremity circulation checks (pulses, temperature, sensation, edema): _pedal pulses 3+ bilaterally, slight edema rt knee and lower leg_ |
|---|---|
| Ted hose/⟨plexi pulses⟩/compression devices: type: _on at all times while in bed_ | Casts, splint, collar, brace: |

**26 CARDIOVASCULAR SYSTEM:** _WNL_

| Pulses (radial, pedal) (to touch or with Doppler): _3+_ | Capillary refill (<3 s): ☒ yes ☐ no | Edema, pitting vs. nonpitting: |
|---|---|---|
| Neck vein (distention): | Sounds: $S_1$, $S_2$, regular, irregular: | Any chest pain: |

**27 RESPIRATORY SYSTEM:** _WNL_

| Depth, rate, rhythm: _20_ | Use of accessory muscles: | Cyanosis: | Sputum: color, amount: | Cough: productive, nonproductive: | Breath sounds: ⟨clear⟩, rales, wheezes: |
|---|---|---|---|---|---|
| Use of oxygen: nasal cannula, mask, trach collar: | Flow rate of oxygen: | Oxygen humidification: ☐ yes ☐ no | Pulse oximeter: _____% oxygen saturation | Smoking: ☒ yes ☐ no | |

**28 GASTROINTESTINAL SYSTEM:** _WNL_

| Abdominal pain, tenderness, guarding; distention ⟨soft⟩ firm: | Bowel sounds x 4 quadrants: _WNL_ | NG tube: describe drainage: |
|---|---|---|
| Ostomy: describe stoma site and stools: | Other: | |

**29 SKIN AND WOUNDS:** _____

| Color, turgor: | Rash, bruises: | Describe wounds (size, location): _surgical incision bruised and edamatous, approximated_ | Edges approximated: ☒ yes ☐ no | Type of wound drains: _Hemovac_ |
|---|---|---|---|---|
| Characteristics of drainage: _red, 50 cc_ | Dressings (clean, dry, intact): _WNL_ | Sutures, staples, steri-strips, other: _sutures intact_ | Risk for decubitus ulcer assessment rating: _20 – low risk_ | Other: |

**30 EYES, EARS, NOSE, THROAT (EENT):** _WNL_

| Eyes: redness, drainage, edema, ptosis | Ears: drainage | Nose: redness, drainage, edema | Throat: sore |
|---|---|---|---|

### PSYCHOSOCIAL AND CULTURAL ASSESSMENT:

| 31 Religious preference (face sheet): | 32 Marital status (face sheet): | 33 Health-care benefits and insurance (face sheet): | 34 Occupation (face sheet): | 35 Emotional state (nurse's notes): |
|---|---|---|---|---|
| _Presbyterian_ | _Married_ | _Aetna_ | _Salesman_ | _Calm, happy surgery is over_ |

#### Additional information to obtain from clinical units the night before clinical specific to your patient's diagnosis:

| Standardized falls-risk assessment: | Pressure ulcer assessment: | Standardized skin assessment: | Standardized nursing care plans: | Clinical pathways: | Patient education materials: |
|---|---|---|---|---|---|
| ☐ yes ☐ no | ☐ yes ☐ no | ☐ yes ☐ no | ☐ yes ☐ no | ☐ yes ☐ no | ☐ yes ☐ no |

■ *Figure* 3–6 *(continued)*

# REFERENCES

1. Standards of Nursing Practice, ed 2. American Nurses Publishing, American Nurses Foundation/ American Nurses Association, Washington, D.C., 1998.
2. Novak, J, and Gowin, DB: Learning How to Learn. Cambridge University Press, New York, 1984.
3. Ausubel, DP, et al: Educational Psychology: A Cognitive View, ed 2. Werbel and Peck, New York, 1986.
4. Deglin, JH, and Vallerand, AH: Davis's Electronic Drug Guide. FA Davis, Philadelphia, 2000.
5. Doenges, ME, et al: Nursing Care Plans: Guidelines for Individualizing Patient Care, ed 5. FA Davis, Philadelphia, 2000.
6. Ibid.
7. Brians, LK, et al: The development of the RISK tool for fall prevention. Rehabilitation Nursing 16(2): 67, 1991.
8. Braden, B, and Bergstrom, N: In Bryant, RA (ed): Acute and Chronic Wounds: Nursing Management. Mosby, St. Louis, 1992.
9. NANDA Nursing Diagnoses: Definitions and Classification, 2001–2002. North American Nursing Diagnosis Association, Philadelphia, 2001.
10. Ibid.
11. Carpenito, LJ: Handbook of Nursing Diagnosis, ed 8. Lippincott, Philadelphia, 1999.
12. Ackley, BJ, and Ladwig, GB: Nursing Diagnosis Handbook, ed 5. Mosby, St. Louis, 2001.
13. Thomas, CL (ed): Taber's Cyclopedic Medical Dictionary, ed 19. FA Davis, Philadelphia, 2001.
14. Sparks, SM, and Taylor, CM: Nursing Diagnosis Reference Manual, ed 5. Springhouse, Springhouse, Pa., 2000.
15. Gordon, M: Manual of Nursing Diagnosis. Including all diagnostic categories approved by the North American Nursing Diagnosis Association. Mosby, St. Louis, 2000.
16. Sparks, SM, and Taylor, CM: Op cit.
17. Gordon, M: Op cit.
18. NANDA: Op cit.
19. Ibid.
20. Ibid.
21. Ibid.
22. Ibid.
23. Ibid.
24. Ibid.

# Chapter 4

## Nursing Interventions:
### So Many Problems, So Little Time

### OBJECTIVES

1. Identify the American Nurses Association Nursing Standards of Clinical Nursing Practice related to identifying patient outcomes and planning nursing interventions.

2. Plan realistic and individualized goals, outcomes, and nursing interventions for each nursing diagnosis.

3. Include individualized physical and psychosocial interventions in each plan of care.

4. Develop an individualized teaching plan for the day of care.

5. Describe the use of information from standardized care plans to selecting typical interventions pertinent to the specific patient assignment on the day of care.

The focus of this chapter is on Step 4 of concept mapping, which involves identifying goals, outcomes, and nursing interventions. The American Nurses Association (ANA) Standards of Clinical Nursing Practice involving outcome identification and planning are standards 3 and 4.[1] ANA standard 3 requires you to identify expected outcomes that must be individualized for your patient. For each nursing diagnosis, you must carefully identify the overall goal and specific patient outcomes. To do that, you need to know the progress that patients typically make in similar situations, and you need to know enough about the specifics of your patient's situation so that you can accurately predict outcomes. Ask yourself, "What will this patient do on the day I'm assigned to care for her to demonstrate that she is making progress and moving toward a healthier state?" Often, patients have multiple problems, and such predictions may become difficult to make. Students commonly grow frustrated because a patient's condition changes between the time they gathered the patient data and the time they arrive on the unit to implement the plan of care. During the interlude, the patient's condition may have changed for better or worse, and the anticipated patient outcomes you created for the day will need to be revised. Sometimes, the patient may have been transferred or even discharged.

Standard 4 mandates that you are responsible for developing a plan of care that prescribes nursing interventions to attain the expected goals and outcomes. You must plan for the patient's physical and emotional care, and you must know what each intervention is intended to accomplish regarding the expected outcomes for the patient. In addition, your plan of care must include development of a specific teaching plan.

The purpose of this chapter is to help develop your critical-thinking process in prioritizing problems, developing patient goals and outcomes, and selecting nursing interventions to attain those goals and outcomes. You will also work on developing a teaching plan for the diabetic patient introduced in earlier chapters.

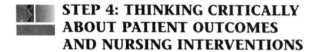

## STEP 4: THINKING CRITICALLY ABOUT PATIENT OUTCOMES AND NURSING INTERVENTIONS

Review the concept map shown in Figure 4–1. It is the one developed in Chapter 3. Note the patient's problem areas: nutrition, urinary elimination, mobility, anxiety, tissue perfusion, and knowledge deficits. Now it is time to arrange these problem areas into priority order.

## Identifying Priority Problem 1

Find the box on the concept map that has the most supporting data in it, and label it Problem No. 1. Usually, the most important diagnosis has the most supporting data and is the priority for planning care. In this example, **Imbalanced Nutrition** is the priority diagnosis. Given the pathophysiology of diabetes mellitus, it makes sense that the patient's nutritional state is going to be highly disrupted, and the patient will need interventions to promote healthy nutrition.

### Assigning Outcomes

As a general goal, the patient would be expected to continue improving his nutritional status. It is important to assess the patient's progress toward this goal and to discern what needs to be accomplished to achieve a healthier state.

For this particular patient, the last known blood glucose level was at 120 mg/dL. Normal blood glucose levels are 80 to 120 mg/dL. Therefore, a major predicted outcome is that the patient will maintain his blood sugar between 80 mg/dL and 120 mg/dL by eating his 1800-calorie diet and taking insulin injections as scheduled.

### Nursing Interventions

What must you do to make sure the patient attains this outcome? The box of data on your concept map gives many clues as to what your interventions will involve:

- Monitor the patient's blood glucose with the Accu-check.
- Monitor the patient's appetite and encourage him to eat his meals.
- Administer his insulin injections as scheduled.
- Watch for signs and symptoms of hypoglycemia, especially if the patient's intake is not sufficient.

You should also monitor the patient for hyperglycemia and obtain a medication order to give additional insulin if indicated.

Take another look at the data in the box for nutrition. What about the polydipsia and 2200-cc intake and 1800-cc output? You will need to continue monitoring the patient's intake and output. Remember that polydipsia and polyuria are classic signs of hyperglycemia, and this patient became dehydrated before he was hospitalized. Currently, his intake exceeds his output because his body is trying to make up for the fluid losses.

The patient's weakness stems from lack of food and from dehydration. Therefore, you will need to monitor his appetite and encourage him to consume his 1800-calorie diet, no sugar added. Calories and food types will need to be carefully regulated against the amount of insulin administered and the patient's level of exercise. Usually, it takes several days of blood glucose monitoring and insulin adjustment before a patient's daily diet, exercise, and insulin patterns can be stabilized. In regulating diabetic patients, it is imperative that there be a counterbalance among calories consumed, insulin dosages, and exercise.

Keep in mind that this patient's weakness is a safety risk. Caution is warranted when transfer-

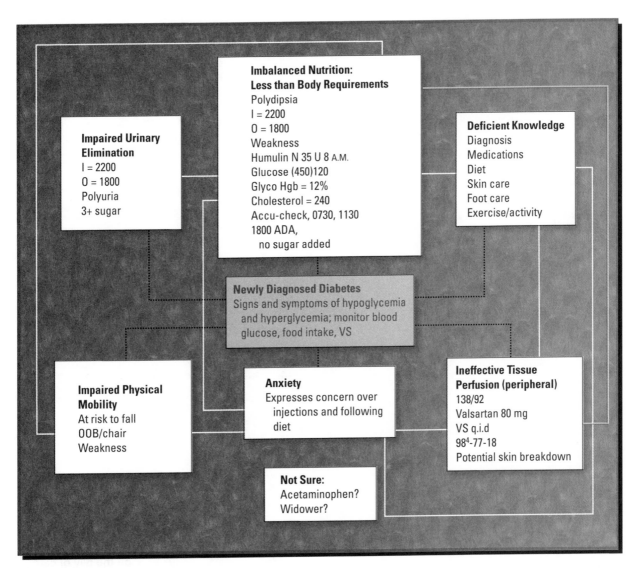

**■■ Figure 4–1**

A completed concept map.

ring him and helping him ambulate. As he continues to progress, he should become stronger. Further assess his weakness level when you first meet him on the day of care by asking him how much help he needs when walking. His risk for falls may also be partly related to his antihypertensive therapy and his age. Antihypertensive drugs commonly cause orthostatic hypotension, which is a drop in blood pressure that causes symptoms of lightheadedness when the patient changes positions, particularly when moved from lying down to sitting or standing up. As people age, the valves inside veins commonly weaken,

which can encourage pooling of blood in the periphery—and which also may result in orthostatic hypotension. To determine the possible effects of orthostatic hypotension on your patient, check his blood pressure and pulse while he sits on the side of his bed. Also, before you help him up, ask him whether he gets dizzy when he stands up. That way, you'll reduce the patient's risk of falling and possibly becoming injured.

The rest of the data in the nutrition box on your concept map addresses additional blood work to check glycohemoglobin (Hgb $A_{1c}$) and cholesterol. These would not be drawn every day.

However, you must plan to check the results of any blood work that is ordered, and promptly report abnormal values to your clinical faculty and the patient's doctor. For example, the doctor may have ordered that electrolytes be drawn. Review those reports as soon as they became available. Always be aware of the time that any blood work is done and the time the reports should be available. Sometimes blood samples get lost. If the reports are not available as scheduled, you may need to contact the laboratory to make sure the blood sample was received and is being processed.

Continuous assessment is indicated when caring for each patient. It is especially important to focus on the primary system of the body affected, in this case, the gastrointestinal system. The basic gastrointestinal (GI) assessment includes bowel sounds, abdominal tenderness, distention, and bowel movements.

**Problem**

Goal:
Behavioral Outcome Objective: The patient will...

on the day of care

| Nursing Interventions | Patient Responses |
| --- | --- |
| 1. | 1. |
| 2. | 2. |
| 3. | 3. |
| 4. | 4. |
| 5. | 5. |
| 6. | 6. |

*Summarize impressions of patient progress toward outcomes:*

**Problem**

Goal:
Behavioral Outcome Objective: The patient will...

on the day of care

| Nursing Interventions | Patient Responses |
| --- | --- |
| 1. | 1. |
| 2. | 2. |
| 3. | 3. |
| 4. | 4. |
| 5. | 5. |
| 6. | 6. |

*Summarize impressions of patient progress toward outcomes:*

■ *Figure* 4–2

Format for writing problems, goals, objectives, interventions, and responses.

## WRITING PROBLEMS, GOALS, OUTCOMES, AND INTERVENTIONS

A blank sample format to guide you in writing out problems, goals, outcomes, and interventions is shown in Figure 4–2. Figure 4–3 contains goals, outcomes, and interventions for the diabetic patient scenario. You have identified nutrition as the top priority for your patient, so write it as Problem No. 1 and list the goals and expected outcomes under this problem. Under the column labeled "Nursing Interventions," write brief notes of all the things you are planning to do, based on what you believe to be important from your analysis of the information in the nutrition box. The right-hand column on the form is reserved for direct observations made of the patient during the clinical day. You will record the patient's responses to each intervention, and

thus use this column to evaluate the patient. This process is explained further in Chapter 5.

The interventions listed so far can be classified as physically supportive of the patient. Nurses "do" physical assessments (GI system), use equipment to monitor patients (Accu-check), monitor laboratory and diagnostic tests (blood glucose), administer medications (insulin), and perform treatments (none for this particular diagnosis).

## ■ Identifying Priority Problem 2

Look back at the concept map again. Anxiety and knowledge deficits are very important interacting diagnoses. The goals are to decrease anxiety and increase knowledge of diabetes. When anxiety is decreased, the patient will be better able to learn, and when he has knowledge of self-care, he will have less anxiety about his ability to perform

---

**Step 4:** Identify goals, outcomes, and interventions

**Problem No. 1** | Imbalanced Nutrition: Less Than Body Requirements

**Goal:** To improve patient's nutritional status
**Outcome:** The patient will maintain blood glucose between 80 and 120 mg/dL by eating his 1800-cal ADA diet and taking insulin injections as scheduled.

| Nursing Interventions | Patient Responses (Evaluation) |
|---|---|
| 1. Check blood glucose with Accu-check at 0800, 1200 | 1. |
| 2. Check for any additional blood work | 2. |
| 3. Assess for s/s of hypoglycemia and hyperglycemia | 3. |
| 4. Monitor oral intake and appetite 1800-cal ADA, no sugar added | 4. |
| 5. Measure fluid intake and output | 5. |
| 6. Give insulin on time | 6. |
| 7. Monitor patient for orthostatic hypotension and weakness | 7. |
| 8. Ambulate patient carefully to avoid falls | 8. |
| 9. Assess abdomen: bowel sounds, tenderness, distention, BMs | 9. |

## ■ Figure 4–3

Step 4. Identifying goals, outcomes, and interventions.

self-care. Anxiety is a common emotional reaction to the stress of illness. For this patient, anxiety may result from his recognition that he must make changes in his lifestyle and that he lacks the confidence and knowledge to make those changes. Consequently, his anxiety must be assessed and reduced before teaching will be successful.

Therefore, anxiety reduction takes priority over patient education. Label it priority Problem No. 2 on your map. Patients are not able to concentrate and learn when anxiety is high. The net result of too much anxiety is usually impaired cognitive function, which simply means that the brain does not work as well. Short-term memory, concentration, and abstract thought can be altered in high-anxiety states. Patients' thoughts are blocked; patients may appear confused and forgetful, and they may have difficulty concentrating. All of these factors contribute to a decreased learning ability. However, a little bit of anxiety can be motivational. If the patient is slightly anxious, his senses are on full alert, and he can use the increased alertness and energy to his advantage to learn about self-care. The goal is to decrease the patient's anxiety but not to completely obliterate it.

The outcome for an anxious patient is to verbalize concerns and express himself. The appropriate interventions are therapeutic communication techniques to facilitate ventilation of feelings and thus relieve the anxiety. Empathy, therapeutic touch, and therapeutic use of humor can be effective techniques to reduce anxiety in this patient situation.

Painful emotions always accompany physical and mental illness. Empathy is a very important communication technique to learn for dealing with patients' painful emotional responses. The classic emotions of sadness, fear, and anger are prevalent during illness. Without release, emotional feelings of sadness can progress to clinical depression; specific fears can progress to diffuse anxiety; and anger may be manifested as hostility and resentment.

Allow the patient to have an emotional release by acknowledging and accepting his emotions and by encouraging him to express those emotions. Do not pretend that his emotions do not exist. Do not criticize emotions. Do not try to rationalize emotions. Do not try to change or fix emotions. At first, the person may yell or blame. He may placate and cry. Or he may be sarcastic and make jokes about his problems. After this period of ventilation, however, he may be able to express his frustrations with his current situation and begin to problem-solve.

Therapeutic touch can be used to decrease the patient's response to anxiety. Carefully monitor the patient's responses to touch. Touch needs to be related to the context of the situation. *Caring touch* includes holding the patient's hand, placing an arm around his shoulders, giving him a hug or a pat on the back. Touch can be used to support, reassure, and raise spirits. *Protective touch* is used where patient safety is a primary concern. A confused patient may be restrained and sedated to make sure he will not pull on vital tubes or fall out of bed. When applying restraints, use caring

| Problem No. 2 | Anxiety | |
|---|---|---|
| | **Goal:** Improve patient's nutritional status **Outcome:** Patient will maintain blood glucose between 70 and 120 mg/dL by eating his 1800-cal ADA diet and taking insulin injections as scheduled. | |
| **Nursing Anxiety Interventions** | | **Patient Responses (Evaluation)** |
| 1. Assess current level of anxiety | | 1. |
| 2. Use empathy | | 2. |
| 3. Use therapeutic touch | | 3. |
| 4. Use therapeutic humor | | 4. |

■ *Figure* 4–4

Anxiety.

touch at the same time. *Task touch* involves physical assessment and procedural treatments that must be done. Be gentle and careful with task touches and overlap them with caring touches.

Therapeutic humor addresses situational dilemmas or points out human weaknesses. Sometimes humor can help to reduce mild anxiety and put people at ease. When people can see the absurdity in a situation and laugh at it, they can distance themselves from threatening problems. Humor is an effective coping mechanism that helps to reframe reality and reduce negative feelings. It facilitates the experience of relief from painful emotions. It is important not to be insulting when using humor and to carefully assess the patient for physical and emotional discomforts before using therapeutic humor.

Based on the above discussion, the problem, goal, outcome, and interventions appear in Figure 4–4 as they would appear on a sample care plan. Additional therapeutic communication techniques are summarized in Box 4–1 and are

---

| **Box 4–1** | *THERAPEUTIC COMMUNICATION TECHNIQUES* |

### Expressions of Sadness and Grief

Tears and crying are very important therapeutic resources that can be used to facilitate healing and well-being. Tears are a natural way of releasing tension that comes from sadness, grief, anger, and fear. Nursing a patient with a loss involves allowing the patient to experience an emotional release through tears. Avoid expressing disapproval or minimizing the cause of crying, and do not offer false hope or make promises that you cannot keep to make the crying stop. Listen supportively and empathetically to patient and family verbalizations of emotional pain.

### Building Self-Esteem

Self-esteem is the value a person places on himself and affects the way he interacts with others. Health problems commonly lower self-esteem. Those with low self-esteem may have feelings of isolation, helplessness, incompetence, or being unloved. To build self-esteem, define clear and realistic goals, help patients to think clearly, give positive feedback, encourage positive self-affirmations, and use visualization exercises.

### Anticipatory Guidance

Nurses use anticipatory guidance to guide patients through uncomfortable procedures. You need to talk to your patients and explain the sensations they will be feeling so they know what to expect and their anxiety will be reduced. For example, when giving an IM injection, say something like, "First I'll palpate and find the right spot. Now you will feel me wiping you off. Now you will feel a pinch and a little burning. It's the medication. All done. I'm massaging the site a little."

### Reminiscing and Life Review

When using reminiscing, the nurse encourages the patient to recall and talk about life experiences. Reminiscing can be helpful in resocializing people and building relationships, while the life review helps people to make sense of their lives and to see their lives as unique stories. Nurses implement reminiscence or life review to help patients deal with crises and losses, to prevent and reduce depression, and to increase life satisfaction.

### Distraction

Distraction is a technique used to take a patient's mind off what is bothering her. The patient may be nervously waiting to have a procedure done. She is prepared for it as well as can be, so you make small talk about whatever interests her. This distraction also works when you are trying to get a slightly confused patient to cooperate with you. For example, say you have a slightly confused elderly patient who is demanding to go for a walk right now, despite having an NG tube, catheters, and IV lines. Although you may need to use light restraints, you may also be able to distract the person from her demand by getting her interested in the television, a magazine, or a conversation.

### Problem-Solving and Decision Making

Nurses commonly help patients solve problems and make decisions. The steps of the problem-solving or decision-making process include identifying the problem, searching for information about the problem, identifying options, examining the pros and cons of each option, choosing an option, developing a plan of action, implementing the plan, and evaluating the effects.

SOURCE: Schuster, P. Communication: The Key to the Therapeutic Relationship. Philadelphia: FA Davis, 2000.

| Problem No. 3 | Deficient Knowledge | |
|---|---|---|
| | **Goal:** Increase knowledge | |
| | **Outcome:** Patient decides in collaboration with the nurse what aspects of diabetic teaching protocol he would like to focus on for the day. | |

| Nursing Education Interventions | Patient Responses (Evaluation) |
|---|---|
| 1. Assess current level of knowledge and establish what the patient most wants to learn about during the day of care. | 1. |
| 2. Assess resources available for teaching such as diabetic educator, dietitian, programs, or movies. | 2. |
| 3. See teaching plan:<br>   —What diabetes is and how it affects health (signs and symptoms)<br>   —Medications<br>   —Diet<br>   —Skin care<br>   —Exercise/activity | 3. |

■ *Figure 4–5*

Deficient Knowledge.

further described in detail in Schuster's *Communication: The Key to the Therapeutic Relationship.*[2]

### ■ Identifying Priority Problem 3

The third priority problem for this patient is deficient knowledge of self-care. Label it as No. 3 on your concept map. It is a nursing responsibility to educate each patient about self-care and to include significant others in your teaching. According to data you have collected for your concept map, this patient is most concerned about injections and diet. One of your first interventions may be to assess his knowledge of injections, diet, and other self-care activities (Figure 4–5). Also ask the nurses what information they have attempted to teach him and how he has responded to their teaching.

As you collected patient data, there was no mention in the patient's records that he had seen a diabetes educator or had attended classes. Find out what resources are available to bridge the gap between what he knows and what he needs to learn. Check to see what types of classes are available to the patient, whether the dietitian has been to talk to him, and whether a diabetes educator is available.

Each patient (and significant other) needs a teaching plan centered on the day of care. This diabetic patient needs to know about his diagno-

sis, medications, diet, exercise, and skin care. He cannot possibly learn all that in one day, but you must develop a general teaching plan before meeting with the patient.

To determine the content of your teaching plan, review a standardized nursing care plan book or computer program for educating patients about major diseases. While obtaining your patient assignment at the health-care agency, get any available teaching aids about his health problems. Read them carefully so you understand the basics of what the patient needs to know. From these resources, pick out the essential teaching information pertinent to your patient. Development of a one-page mini-individualized teaching plan with specific content and teaching methods is the focus of the last section of this chapter.

### ■ Identifying Priority Problem 4

Review your concept map and look at the remaining diagnoses to select the problem of the fourth priority. The box with the diagnosis **Ineffective Tissue Perfusion (peripheral)** contains more information, so you can label it Problem No. 4. The pathophysiology of diabetes affects the circulation; many diabetics have a history of hypertension. Specifically, diabetes speeds up degeneration of the arteries and veins, and fat

| Problem No. 4 | Ineffective Tissue Perfusion (peripheral) | |
|---|---|---|

**Goal:** Maintain optimal tissue perfusion and circulation

**Outcome:** Vital signs remain close to normal, no skin breakdown. Patient gets up at least twice, sits in a chair, and does range-of-motion exercises with additional walking with assistance if able.

| Nursing Tissue Perfusion Interventions | Patient Responses (Evaluation) |
|---|---|
| 1. Monitor VS q4h | 1. |
| 2. Give atenolol, check BP/P before administration | 2. |
| 3. Chair x 2 | 3. |
| 4. ROM extremities q2h if in bed | 4. |
| 5. Walk w/ assistance if able | 5. |
| 6. Assess skin for ulcers | 6. |

■ *Figure 4–6*

Inefficient Tissue Perfusion.

deposits build up in the blood vessels, leading to atherosclerosis and hypertension. Atherosclerosis is the cause of coronary artery disease (heart attacks), cerebral vascular disease (strokes), and peripheral vascular disease (hypertension). Peripheral vascular disease has many implications for diabetics. With inadequate tissue perfusion, tissues will break down and pressure ulcers will form. Nerve degeneration also occurs in the periphery. This is termed *diabetic neuropathy* and results in pain, tingling, and burning in the legs. Neuropathy progresses to a lack of sensation in the legs as the disease worsens.

Therefore, the general goal would be to maintain optimal tissue perfusion and circulation (Figure 4–6). Specific outcomes include keeping the patient's vital signs close to normal and avoiding skin breakdown. You will be monitoring his vital signs and assessing his circulation by checking capillary refill and peripheral pulses. You will also watch for skin ulcers, encourage supervised ambulation, help the patient into a chair, and encourage him to perform range-of-motion exercises to improve circulation to his limbs and prevent skin breakdown.

## ■ Identifying Priority Problems 5 and 6

The two remaining diagnoses that have not been directly addressed include **Impaired Physical Mobility** and **Impaired Urinary Elimination**. These diagnoses are of equal importance and have been labeled Problems No. 5 and No. 6 on the concept map. It doesn't matter which is Problem 5 and which is Problem 6, as long as both are recognized as problems.

The goal for **Impaired Physical Mobility** is to prevent complications of immobility and to prevent falls. The patient outcomes are to sit in a chair with assistance, to perform range-of-motion exercises, and to ambulate as much as tolerated. Interventions to attain these outcomes have been covered in Problems 1 and 4. Specifically, you will monitor the patient for orthostatic hypotension and weakness, and you will carefully assist the patient with ambulation to avoid falls. You will also help the patient sit in a chair and perform range-of-motion exercises.

The goal for **Impaired Urinary Elimination** is to maintain normal urinary elimination. Outcomes include intake and output approaching normal values, and that the patient has no polyuria. Interventions are covered under Problem 1 and include measuring fluid intake and output and monitoring for signs and symptoms of hyperglycemia and hypoglycemia.

The goals and outcomes for **Impaired Physical Mobility** and **Impaired Urinary Elimination** are shown Figure 4–7. There is no need to copy interventions that you have already specified into this summary. Instead, refer to the

| Problem No. 5 | Impaired Physical Mobility | |
|---|---|---|
| | **Goal:** Prevent complications of immobility and prevent falls | |
| | **Outcome:** Patient ambulates to chair and walks if able, otherwise does range-of-motion exercises | |
| **Nursing Mobility Interventions** | | **Patient Responses (Evaluation)** |
| Covered under nutrition and altered tissue perfusion | | |

| Problem No. 6 | Impaired Urinary Mobility | |
|---|---|---|
| | **Goal:** Maintain normal urinary elimination | |
| | **Outcome:** Intake and output approaching normal values, no polyuria | |
| **Nursing Urinary Elimination Interventions** | | **Patient Responses (Evaluation)** |
| Covered under nutrition | | |

■ *Figure 4–7*

Impaired Physical Mobility.

interventions covered under previous nursing diagnoses.

Your basic care plan is now complete. You can carry the concept map, complete with goals, outcomes, interventions, and teaching plan, in your pocket on the clinical units and use it during the implementation phase of the nursing process. Be prepared to discuss with your clinical faculty the rationales for each of the interventions you identified. Although the basic care plan is complete, you still need to develop a teaching plan. What follows is a discussion of one method for developing a teaching plan.

 **DEVELOPING A MINI–TEACHING PLAN**

Box 4–2 shows an outline that you can use to develop a one-page mini–teaching plan. This outline focuses on key information that all patients and significant others need to know about their specific disease and its treatments. The key teaching areas are structured around the acronym METHOD.[3,4]

Using a specific method to teach content (in this case, the acronym) will help you remember key items to cover in every teaching plan you construct. Teaching is an essential component of all care planning. Students are required to come to clinical prepared to teach whatever is appropriate for the clinical day. If you are assigned to a preoperative patient, focus on preoperative teaching. If you are assigned to a first-day surgical patient, focus teaching on the first day after surgery. Focus on discharge teaching if the patient is being prepared to go home while you are taking care of him.

■ **Completing the METHOD Teaching Plan**

**M IS FOR MEDICATIONS**

Write the name (generic and brand name) and key action for each drug. Write one sentence for each drug that represents how you would explain it to your patient in words the patient and significant others can understand. Avoid using medical terminology from your drug guides. Use medical terminology only when explaining a drug's actions and side effects to your clinical faculty as you are preparing the drugs for administration. For example, write:

- "This is an antibiotic for your infection."
- "This is a blood thinner to prevent clots."
- "This is your pain pill."
- "This is your insulin to control your blood sugar."

Details about side effects are not necessary unless the patient is going home with the drug or is

## Box 4–2    METHOD FORMAT FOR DEVELOPING A TEACHING PLAN

**Patient Name:**

**Diagnosis:**

**Teaching Techniques:**

M (Medications)

E (Environment)

T (Treatments)

H (Health knowledge of disease)

O (Outpatient/inpatient referrals)

D (Diet)

asking for more specific information. If he's going home with the drug, write the basics of what you will say in simple terms with as few words as possible. For example, "Take Tylenol (acetaminophen) if you need something for discomfort. Don't take aspirin because it is a blood thinner" or "Take your antibiotic three times a day: when you get up, in the afternoon, and at night before bed. Take the entire prescription. Don't stop before it's finished, even if you feel better. Take it with food if your stomach gets upset."

### E IS FOR ENVIRONMENT

Environment includes home or health-care agency environment, financial considerations, and social support. Review standardized nursing care plan guides and nursing texts to determine how the patient and his significant others may need to modify the home environment. Assess the patient's home situation and intervene if needed. Determine whether the patient has the financial resources to implement the treatment plan, and intervene if necessary. Find out whether the patient has significant others to assist with care if needed. Contacts with community agencies may be necessary to assist in the adjustment to returning home if significant others are not available. Also consider what you must do to provide a safe environment in the health-care setting.

### T IS FOR TREATMENTS

Explain the purpose of each treatment and the correct techniques for performing treatments that will continue at home. For example, explain skin care procedures or wound care. Write down specifically what the patient needs to do. If written guidelines are available, highlight the most important things for the patient to remember. Exercise or activity guidelines may also be considered a treatment. Each patient must be aware of activities that are and are not permitted, and how to develop and maintain an exercise routine. Many diabetic patients will be instructed to gradually increase their walking until they are walking for 30 minutes four or more days a week.

### H IS FOR HEALTH KNOWLEDGE OF DISEASE

Write down the effects of the patient's disease, signs and symptoms that he should watch for,

and any changes that should prompt him to call the physician. For example, write down what the patient should watch for regarding signs and symptoms of an infection in a wound, a urine infection, or whatever is applicable to the specific patient problems.

### O IS FOR OUTPATIENT/INPATIENT REFERRALS

Write a sentence to explain inpatient diagnostic tests or procedures using nonmedical terms. For outpatient referrals, list support groups, home health agencies, office appointments, and any pertinent dates and times. Check with the staff nurses during your assigned clinical day to find out the physician's usual routine for patients after discharge. Also, read the discharge orders.

### D IS FOR DIET

Write down the patient's appropriate diet and restrictions. Obtain examples of typical menus from the dietitian. Write down a list of foods that the patient can eat and foods that he should avoid as applicable.

## ■ Sample METHOD Plan for a Diabetic Patient

For the diabetic patient in Figure 4–1, the METHOD teaching plan will result from a synthesis of concept map data, standardized teaching plans, and patient education materials for diabetic patients. You will need to review a standardized teaching plan for diabetics, standardized insulin patient information, standardized 1800-calorie (American Diabetic Association) ADA diet samples, and patient education booklets on diabetes. The following section walks you through the construction of a METHOD teaching plan for this patient.

### MEDICATIONS

Three drugs are listed on your concept map: Humulin N, valsartan, and acetaminophen. Based on information you glean from drug references, your patient teaching information about the patient's medications may look something like what appears in Box 4–3. It is formatted using the actual words you might say to the patient.

## Box 4–3 *METHOD DAILY TEACHING PLAN*

**Patient Initials:** E. T.

**Diagnosis:** Newly diagnosed diabetes

### Medications

Humulin N (NPH, human insulin) insulin: "This drug is to control blood glucose levels. Watch for signs and symptoms of hypoglycemia and hyperglycemia. Onset (1 to 2 hours), peak (6 to 12 hours) and duration (up to 24 hours). Take this drug each morning 30 minutes before breakfast. If you do not eat as scheduled and in the amounts specified in your diet plan, you will probably have a hypoglycemic reaction in mid- to late afternoon (6 to 12 hours after you've taken the drug)."

Valsartan (Diovan): "This drug is to control your blood pressure. Watch for signs of low blood pressure. Get up slowly and sit on the side of the bed to avoid dizziness. Check your blood pressure and pulse."

Acetaminophen (Tylenol): "Take this drug in recommended amounts for aches and general discomfort; don't take aspirin because aspirin causes blood thinning and could upset your stomach."

### Environment

Assess patient for social supports to help him with self-care and transportation. Teach patient activity limitations while the patient is in the hospital, and find out activity prescription after discharge. Create an environment of trust and support so the patient can learn effectively.

### Treatments

Demonstrate use of Accu-check or have patient do procedure if ready. Use patient teaching aid booklet and video if available.

Demonstrate insulin injection or have patient self-administer if ready. Demonstrate care of equipment. Use patient teaching aid booklet and video if available.

Describe skin care, wound care (if appropriate), and daily care of feet using teaching aids such as booklets or videos. Highlight information in patient teaching pamphlets: Use mild soap and lukewarm water. Use lotions to keep skin soft. Protect skin by using gloves while working and sunscreen while outdoors. Treat injuries immediately with soap, warm water, and dry sterile bandage. See physician or nurse practitioner if cuts do not heal or become infected (red, throbbing, warm, swelling, pus).

Explain activity limitations and have patient reiterate. "You will be out of bed to sit in a chair and walk with assistance today. Until your strength returns, you will need assistance to prevent falls."

### Health Knowledge of Disease

"Hypoglycemia may be caused by taking in too much insulin, missing or delaying meals, exercising or working more than usual, or getting an infection or illness. It can develop rapidly, in 15 minutes to 1 hour. Symptoms include sweating, dizziness, shaking, hunger, or restlessness; numbness/tingling of the lips, tongue, hands, or feet; slurred speech, headache, or blurred vision. Carry candy or fruit juice with you and drink it if you feel a hypoglycemic reaction coming. When the reaction is over, eat a serving of a slowly digested food such as cottage cheese, milk, or your scheduled meal or snack to prevent a second drop in blood sugar."

"Hyperglycemia can be caused by omitting insulin or taking less than prescribed, eating more than the prescribed diet, or experiencing a great deal of stress. Illnesses with fever and infection may also cause hyperglycemia. Diabetic acidosis can result over a period of hours or days. You had symptoms of hyperglycemia before coming into the hospital; they included excessive urination and thirst. You were tired, you lost weight, and you were dehydrated. Other signs and symptoms of hyperglycemia may include drowsiness, loss of appetite, blurred vision, abdominal pain, nausea, vomiting, and a fruity odor to your breath. To avoid hyperglycemia, follow your meal plan closely, test your blood glucose levels regularly, and report any consistently high levels. Call for an appointment with your physician or nurse practitioner when you have a fever or when a wound looks like it could be infected."

### Outpatient/Inpatient Tests/Referrals

Sequential blood glucose monitoring: "The purpose of doing fingersticks with the Accu-check before meals and at bedtime is to determine if the insulin and food you are taking is in the correct balance to control your blood glucose levels."

Provide local and national resources.

### Diet

1800-calorie ADA diet, no added sugar. Attach sample menu and exchange lists. Include significant others in teaching meal planning and following exchange lists.

Keep in mind that although this section of the teaching plan is written to the patient, the plan is actually for your use and not to be given to the patient. Naturally, you should be prepared to discuss the details of your teaching plan with your clinical faculty before giving a drug or even giving the patient this information. You should also be prepared to give the patient more information if he asks for it.

## ENVIRONMENT

Your patient is an 80-year-old widower. He has insurance. To fill out this section of the teaching plan, assess him further to find out about his level of social support. Does he have family members or significant others to assist him at home and take him to follow-up appointments or diabetic education classes? Does he drive? While in the hospital, what special assistance did he need in his environment that he will still need at home? For example, he needs to be carefully assisted with ambulation until his strength returns. He needs to be taught his activity restrictions while hospitalized. Therefore, the teaching plan could include the notations included in Box 4–3 listed under Environment.

## TREATMENTS

The patient, someone in his family, or another person must learn to use the Accu-check device, draw up and give insulin, and keep records of the patient's blood glucose levels and the amount of insulin administered. Including these items on your teaching plan would look something like what appears in Box 4–3 under Treatments. Give the patient written instructions for how to use the Accu-check and how to administer insulin. As you demonstrate how to check blood glucose levels and give an insulin injection, provide simple instructions for each step. Then ask the patient to give you a return demonstration, in which he tries to use the Accu-check and give himself an insulin injection. Reassure him and help him; he will be anxious at first.

Also, explain and demonstrate what the patient needs to do to care for his skin and feet. Again, have him give you a return demonstra-

tion. If the patient's nurse has already taught him these skills, check his understanding by asking him questions or watching him demonstrate them.

## HEALTH KNOWLEDGE OF DISEASE

The patient needs to know the signs and symptoms of his disease and when it is time to call the physician or nurse practitioner. In this case, it is most important for the patient to know about hypoglycemia and hyperglycemia and what to do about these conditions when they occur. Review the signs and symptoms of hypoglycemia and hyperglycemia with the patient, and explain the circumstances most likely to precipitate symptoms. Again, consult Box 4–3 under Health Knowledge of Disease for an example of what your teaching plan might say.

## INPATIENT AND OUTPATIENT REFERRALS

Be prepared to explain any test or procedure in a sentence or two using nonmedical terminology. This particular patient is not scheduled for any blood tests in addition to his blood glucose levels. But be prepared to explain when, where, how, and why sequential blood glucose tests are needed as applicable to the patient situation, as described in Box 4–3 under Outpatient/Inpatient Referrals.

There is no way to predict what other tests will be ordered, and you are not expected to memorize every single test. The more common tests will become very familiar as your experiences and knowledge increase. There will always be references available to look up laboratory tests and procedures on your unit. You can also call the laboratory or department in which the test is being done and ask them to give you patient information materials for the particular test or procedure that your patient is to have.

It is helpful to give patients information on local and national resources concerning their health problems. The Internet is an excellent resource to locate addresses or phone numbers of agencies so that patients and their significant others have a place to start looking for more information if they are interested. For example, national diabetes resources include:

- American Diabetes Association National Service Center, 1660 Duke Street, Alexandria VA 22314 or 1-800-DIABETES (1-800-342-2383) or on the Internet at
  *http://www.diabetes.org/default.htm*
- Diabetes resources on the Internet
  *http://vigora.com/resources/*
- National Diabetes Information Clearinghouse, 1 Information Way, Bethesda MD 20892-3560 or on the Internet at
  *http://www.niddk.nih.gov/health/diabetes/ndic.htm*

Once you know what the national organizations are, look in the phone book to determine whether there is a local branch of the organization. If so, provide the patient or significant other with the appropriate phone numbers.

At this point in your planning process, you have no specific data about the patient's discharge. However, the physician or nurse practitioner will provide instructions for scheduling follow-up appointments and arranging for a home health-care agency, if necessary.

### DIET

This patient has been prescribed an 1800-calorie ADA diet with no added sugar. You will need to teach him now to use a food exchange list. Fruits, breads, meats, fats, and milk products are grouped in lists. Exchange lists and sample menus may be obtained from the dietary department in the health-care agency. You can also call the American Dietetic Association at 1-800-366-1655. Online information is available at the Web site *www.eatright.org*.

Plan to sit down with the patient to discuss the diet and the food lists. Ask him to plan his meals according to what he likes to eat, using the exchange lists. Plan to have significant others also hear your instructions, especially the person who usually prepares the patient's meals.

The preceding discussion of the teaching plan includes details of teaching content and rationales. Using Box 4–2 as a guide your mini-teaching plan should be no more than about one page long. It should provide an outline of what you will need to implement. Attach all relevant teaching materials you will be using. There is no need to rewrite and duplicate information found in the teaching materials and standardized care plans.

In summary, the METHOD daily teaching plan is a focused, individualized plan based on data from the concept maps and general standardized teaching plans. You are expected to attach relevant teaching materials to the plan.

### ■ Developing Teaching Skills

To be an effective teacher, you must know not only what to teach but also how to teach it. Most importantly, you must assess the patient and significant others for learning readiness before trying to teach anything. For example, if the patient is highly anxious or in considerable pain, or if he's tired or hungry, you may try to teach him something; however, chances are that he'll retain little of the information you provide, and he may become more anxious besides.

To teach effectively, you will need to use basic principles of teaching and learning in adults and children, and you will need to use learning principles, teaching strategies, and evaluation methods (Box 4–4). For further discussion of basic principles of learning and teaching strategies, refer to Chapter 9 in *Communication: The Key to the Therapeutic Relationship* by Schuster.[2] Therapeutic communication is the foundation of the nurse-patient relationship. You must know how to use therapeutic communication throughout the process of teaching.

In conclusion, teaching plans focus on data from the concept map and on general patient teaching information prioritized to address the most important problems first. Keep in mind that anxiety blocks communication and learning and that even a calm patient can only absorb so much information at one time. Where possible, ask the patient where he would like to start, and then be flexible. Bring your detailed standardized care plans with you and refer to them if the patient asks questions you are not prepared to answer. Students are not expected to know every aspect of teaching about every health problem. As needed, refer questions to your clinical faculty, staff nurses, or, in this case, to a diabetes educator.

---

**Box 4-4** | **ADULT LEARNING PRINCIPLES**

Use these principles when teaching adult patients:

- Build on previous experiences.
- Focus on immediate concerns first.
- Adapt teaching to the patient's lifestyle.
- Make the patient an active participant.
- Determine learning readiness.
- Be realistic and stick to the basics.
- Take advantage of the teachable moment by incorporating teaching into your ongoing patient care.
- Reinforce all learning.
- Solicit feedback.

**Knowledge-Based Teaching Strategies**

Your teaching methods must coincide with the type of knowledge you are trying to convey. Use these techniques:

- *Cognitive knowledge (facts):* Give explanations and descriptions. Use books, pamphlets, films, programmed instruction, and computer programs.
- *Affective and cognitive knowledge (feelings and beliefs):* Use one-to-one discussions, group discussions, role-playing, and discovery to guide the patient in problem-solving situations that help him express feelings and use cognitive knowledge to solve problems.
- *Psychomotor knowledge (skills):* Use demonstrations accompanied by explanations.

**Evaluation of Teaching:
Did the Patient Learn?**

To assess your patient's learning, use these techniques.

- *Cognitive knowledge:* Ask oral or written questions. Ask the patient to keep a diary or records of self-monitoring.
- *Affective knowledge:* Infer the patient's level of learning from how he responds to you, how he speaks about his illness and his treatments, and how he verbally expresses his feelings and values.
- *Psychomotor knowledge:* Ask the patient for a return demonstration.

---

## CHAPTER SUMMARY

The purpose of this chapter was to guide you in the development of Step 4 of the concept map care planning process. Step 4 involves developing goals, outcomes, and nursing interventions for each diagnosis. Nursing interventions are developed to physically support patients and to provide the services that patients cannot provide for themselves. Nursing interventions are also intended to provide psychosocial support.

Step 4 is based on thinking critically and synthesizing information from standardized care plans and the data available on the concept map. Step 4 also involves developing a teaching plan for the patient and significant others. The components of the teaching plan for the day of care can be remembered using the acronym METHOD. These letters stand for the key elements of a teaching plan: medications, environment, treatments, health knowledge, outpatient/inpatient tests/referrals, and diet.

Carry your concept map, goals, outcomes, interventions, and teaching plan in your pocket on the clinical unit. Also, bring the standardized care plans, clinical pathways (if available), medication cards or printouts, and relevant patient education teaching materials as needed. In addition, bring the patient profile database with the falls-risk assessment and pressure ulcer risk scale. What you need to bring to the clinical site is listed in Box 4–5.

| **Box 4–5** | *CHECKLIST: WHAT TO BRING TO THE CLINICAL AGENCY* |
|---|---|

1. Patient profile database
2. Concept map based on patient profile database (Steps 1–3)
3. Plan of Goals/Outcomes/Interventions (Step 4)
4. Pressure ulcer risk assessment scale
5. Falls-risk assessment scale
6. METHOD teaching plan
7. Patient education materials
8. Standardized care plans
9. Clinical pathways, if available
10. Printouts or medication cards for all drugs

## LEARNING ACTIVITIES

To do these exercises, you will need access to books on medical-surgical nursing, nutrition, medications, diagnostic tests and procedures, and standardized care plans. One approach is to form a group ahead of time and have each person bring a specific reference to class instead of having each student carry in all their own references.

1. Work in groups of three to four students to develop Step 4 goals, outcomes, and interventions for patient Scenarios 2 and 3, which appear in the end-of-chapter exercises for Chapter 3. Split up the diagnoses among the groups. Each group should write its goals, outcomes, and interventions on the board for critique by the entire class.

2. A representative of each group should state rationales for the interventions for the assigned diagnosis.

3. Develop METHOD teaching plans for patient Scenarios 2 and 3. Split up the components of the teaching plan (tests, environment, treatments, health knowledge, outpatient/inpatient referrals, and diet) among the group. Write the teaching components on the board so the entire class can critique the content of the teaching plan.

4. A representative of each group should state the teaching methods and evaluation techniques that would be used to teach the information.

5. Using the diabetic patient in this chapter as an example, explain what you would say and do to assess his anxiety, show empathy, and use therapeutic touch and therapeutic humor.

## REFERENCES

1. Standards of Nursing Clinical Practice, ed 2. American Nurses Publishing, American Nurses Foundation/American Nurses Association, Washington, D.C., 1998.
2. Schuster, PM: Communication: The Key to the Therapeutic Relationship. FA Davis, Philadelphia, 2000.
3. Ibid.
4. Huey, R, et al: Discharge planning: Good planning means fewer hospitalizations for the chronically ill. Nursing 81, 11–20, 1981.

# Chapter 5

## Nursing Implementation:
### Using Concept Map Care Plans in the Health-Care Agency

## OBJECTIVES

1. Describe clinical organizational strategies necessary for successful clinical performance.

2. Identify American Nurses Association (ANA) Standards of Clinical Practice related to implementation and evaluation of nursing care plans in the health-care agency.

3. Describe how to update and modify a concept map care plan on arrival to the clinical agency.

4. Relate how to use a concept map care plan during interactions with patients.

5. Describe the evaluation of patient responses to nursing interventions done during Step 5 of the concept map care planning process.

6. Describe how the map can be used to facilitate communication between the student nurse, the clinical faculty, and the staff nurse.

7. Use the concept map to explain the relationship between medications and relevant clinical data before giving drugs.

8. Describe the development of concept maps for use in outpatient settings.

The concept map care plan is used as an organizational tool for clinical data. A focus of this chapter is on organizational strategies to prioritize what must be done during a clinical day. This chapter also describes implementation and evaluation of nursing care using the concept map care plan.

Standard 5 of the ANA Standards of Clinical Nursing Practice mandates that nurses are responsible for the implementation of interventions identified in the nursing care plan.[1] In the clinical setting, the concept map care plan becomes a dynamic working clinical tool to assist you with organizing the data for the ongoing care of your patients. You need to be able to update the plan to account for dynamic changes that regularly occur in clinical settings. You will face many challenges throughout a clinical day. Nothing ever goes exactly as planned!

The final criterion of the ANA Standards of Clinical Nursing Practice is standard 6, which states that nurses must take responsibility for evaluating patients' progress toward attaining their outcomes and goals.[2] This is accomplished by identifying patient responses to interventions, which is Step 5 of the concept map care plan. You must discipline yourself to carefully focus on and evaluate patient responses to each intervention, and you must record these responses on the concept map care plan.

 ## ARRIVAL IN THE INPATIENT UNIT: GETTING ORGANIZED

Getting organized is crucial for successful clinical performance. When you arrive at the clinical unit, you must obtain the latest data for medications, intravenous fluids, and treatments along with a patient status report. Write updates directly on your concept map care plan. Put new data on the diagram under the appropriate diagnoses. Do not use a separate sheet of paper for the updates because a separate sheet of paper could easily get lost. Use a red pen so you and your clinical faculty can quickly see your revisions. A prioritized list of all the activities you must complete to update your plan of care is shown in Box 5–1.

### ▄▄ Check Medication Records

Check for changes in the patient's medications by reviewing medication records for routine and p.r.n. (for emergency, as needed) drugs. Update your concept map by adding, deleting, or revising drugs. Write the times at which medications

should be administered on the front of the map in red ink. Highlight medications so you can find them easily on the map.

Write down on the map what time the patient last received a p.r.n. pain medication, along with the name of the drug. If you are not familiar with any of the drugs the patient is receiving, you will need to either look them up in a drug reference book or call the pharmacy to obtain drug information before giving the medication.

### ▄▄ Check IV Administration Records

Check for changes in the patient's IV records. Write down the current fluid being administered and rate of administration on the concept map diagram in the appropriate nursing diagnosis box. Highlight the intravenous fluid and rate of administration. Also note and highlight admixtures and length of infusion time.

### ▄▄ Check Treatments

Check for updates in the patient's treatments and write these on the concept map in the appropriate nursing diagnosis box. If the data does not fit in any of the diagnostic boxes that appear on the map, then you will need to make a new diagnosis box. If you aren't sure where the new information goes, place it in a corner box and check with your clinical faculty.

### ▄▄ Check Laboratory Data

Check the records for laboratory tests and diagnostic procedures that were ordered from the time you left the unit. Find out which laboratory tests and procedures were completed and which reports are pending. For completed laboratory tests and procedures, find the reports and write the results on your concept map in the appropri-

| **Box 5–1** | **WHAT TO DO WHEN YOU ARRIVE AT THE UNIT** |
|---|---|
| 1. Check the patient's medication record. | 4. Check the patient's laboratory data. |
| 2. Check the patient's IV administration record. | 5. Obtain a patient report from the off-going shift. |
| 3. Check the patient's treatments. | |

ate diagnostic categories. For pending laboratory results, write in the name of the test and place a blank next to it so you will know to fill in the result when it becomes available. Typically, the daily morning blood work is drawn between 5 and 6 A.M., and laboratory reports come back to the units early. You must have the latest information on laboratory data before administering many of the patient's drugs. For example, if you need to give Lanoxin (digoxin) and Lasix (furosemide), you will first need to know the most recent potassium value.

It is also crucial to analyze blood samples that are related to medications because side effects of medications are often detected through analysis of blood samples. In this example, Lasix causes potassium to be lost in the urine. Hypokalemia may result in digitalis toxicity.

### ▇ Obtain Information from the Previous Shift

There is always an end-of-shift summary report for each patient. It is crucial for you to obtain a report of the patient's recent health status. Change-of-shift reports may take many different forms, including:

- A verbal report with all oncoming nursing staff taking notes on all patients
- Tape-recorded reports
- Written reports
- Verbal one-on-one reports between the nurse who is leaving and the nurse who is starting to deliver care to a particular group of patients

Write the information you obtain from the change-of-shift report in the appropriate nursing diagnosis boxes on your map. Or, if necessary, make a new box if the data suggests a new nursing diagnosis. If you don't know where new information belongs on your map, put it in a corner box and check with your clinical faculty.

In short, as soon as you get to the health-care agency, you will need to start collecting data to update your concept map care plan. Obtain data from medication records, IV records, treatments, laboratory data, and staff nurses. Don't forget to look at the laboratory data that was collected while you were gone, and note any laboratory

data that is pending. Medications are usually the priority; many (such as insulin and Lasix) must be given on time. It is also important to give pain medications on time. So always check medications before anything else, because you may need to give a medication before doing anything else.

The nurses at the end of their shifts will be busy finishing up their documentation and preparing their reports for the oncoming shift. This is not a good time to ask them questions. The outgoing nurses will give you and the oncoming nurses a shift report as scheduled when they've completed their work. After the shift report, you may ask them additional questions before they leave.

 ### CLINICAL PRECONFERENCE

For many students, a clinical preconference is held early in the clinical day, after the change-of-shift report. The purpose of the preconference is for clinical faculty to meet with students to review the accuracy of the plans of care. By looking at your map, your clinical faculty will be able to see very quickly if you have collected, correctly analyzed, and categorized adequate data. Goals, outcomes, and interventions can also be reviewed quickly. The succinct lists on a concept map facilitate a rapid evaluation of the plan of care.

You must be prepared to orally address questions concerning your plan of care. This includes assessment data, nursing and medical diagnoses, goals, outcomes, interventions, and rationales. After the preconference, keep the concept map in your pocket to guide you throughout the day.

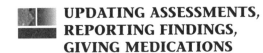 ### UPDATING ASSESSMENTS, REPORTING FINDINGS, GIVING MEDICATIONS

After determining your initial priorities and completing your preconference, you will need to accomplish several more specific tasks (Box 5–2). They include patient assessment, reporting the findings of your assessment, and preparing to give medications.

| Box 5–2 | WHAT TO DO AFTER UPDATING THE CARE PLAN |
|---------|------------------------------------------|

1. Perform patient assessment.

2. Report assessment data to patient's assigned staff nurse.

3. Report assessment data to clinical faculty.

4. Locate medications.

5. Meet faculty in medication area to prepare for drug administration (if applicable).

## Patient Assessment and Evaluation

If the patient is sleeping, wake him to do your first assessment of the clinical day. If you are like many beginning students, you may not want to disturb the patient's sleep. However, it is critical that you have the assessment data you need to make sound clinical judgments. In fact, it's possible that the patient isn't sleeping at all but comatose, and you wouldn't know that unless you attempted to rouse him. A diabetic patient could be unconscious from hypoglycemia. It is a professional standard of care that assessments are done on each patient early at the start of each shift. Write your findings in the evaluation column of your care plan, shown in Figure 5–1. The recorded notes of patient responses are the fifth step of the concept map care plan.

## Reporting Assessment Data

Once you have done your assessment and evaluation and have taken notes, you need to quickly find your patient's assigned staff nurse, introduce yourself if necessary, and report your assessment findings. If you see your clinical faculty before you see the patient's nurse, report your findings to the clinical faculty first. You must report to both of them early in the shift.

Once the patient's immediate needs are met, you need to review with the patient's assigned staff nurse what you will and will not be doing for patient care. You may need to say, "I don't know how to do the dressing change yet" or "I can't do the Accu-check." The staff nurse is responsible for doing what you have not yet learned to do, so you must be very clear about what you can do and what she will need to do. She may review the daily plan of care with you,

emphasizing the important aspects of care that must be done from her viewpoint.

If you meet with the patient's staff nurse first, tell your clinical faculty as soon as you're finished. Likewise, if you report to your clinical faculty first, find the patient's staff nurse as soon as you're done. Communication must flow openly between you, the faculty, and the patient's staff nurse. Assessment and patient evaluation involves critical information that both your faculty and patient's assigned staff nurse want to know as soon as possible during the first hour of the shift.

Any time you find abnormalities in any of your patient's assessment data, interrupt the staff nurse or your clinical faculty to report the abnormality. The key words here are *interrupt* and *any abnormalities*. Abnormalities include anything not within normal parameters. For example, a blood pressure of 150/92 is not within normal parameters. Many students hesitate to interrupt when the faculty or staff nurses look busy. However, do not wait until the faculty or staff nurse appears to be free. Get the attention of one or the other no matter how busy they might appear. Abnormal assessment data means the patient could be getting into trouble, and the staff nurse and clinical faculty have the knowledge to make a clinical judgment about what is an imminent danger and what can wait until later. Each of these nurses will want to further assess and evaluate the patient's responses.

Even if you find and interrupt your clinical faculty and she tells you that she can't come to the patient's bedside immediately, she will tell you to find the patient's assigned staff nurse or the charge nurse. She will check on you and your patient as soon as possible. If the staff nurse and clinical faculty are both too busy, they will refer you to yet another nurse.

| Step 4: | Identify goals, outcomes, and interventions | Step 5: | Evaluate patient responses |

**Problem No. 1**    **Imbalanced Nutrition**

**Goal:** Improve patient's nutritional status
**Outcome:** Patient will maintain blood glucose between 70 and 120 mg/dL by eating his 1800-cal ADA diet and taking insulin injections as scheduled.

| Step 4 Nursing Nutrition Interventions Step | Step 5 Patient Responses (Evaluation) |
| --- | --- |
| 1. Check blood glucose with Accu-check at 0800, 1200 | 1. 60 at 7:30, 100 at 11:30 |
| 2. Check for any additional blood work | 2. 6:00 electrolytes pending K = 3.8 |
| 3. Assess for s/s of hypoglycemia and hyperglycemia | 3. 7:45 sweaty, dizzy, hungry |
| 4. Check to make sure patient eats 1800-cal ADA, no sugar added | 4. Ate 90% breakfast, 50% lunch |
| 5. Measure intake and output | 5. I = 400, 350, 200 O = 250, 225, 300 |
| 6. Give insulin on time. | 6. 8:00 insulin held, Dr. notified Continue Accu-check and call for further orders after each Accu-check |
| 7. Monitor patient for orthostatic hypotension and weakness | 7. Steady while standing and walking BP = 124/60 standing up |
| 8. Ambulate patient carefully to avoid falls | 8. Able to walk without assistance to BR |
| 9. Assess abdomen: bowel sounds, tenderness, distension, BMs | 9. BS all quads |

*Impressions: Need to continue to carefully monitor for hypoglycemia and hyperglycemia because diet, insulin, and blood sugar still not coordinated. Is stronger and is cautious with movement.*

**Problem No. 2**    **Anxiety**

**Goal:** Improve patient's nutritional status
**Outcome:** Patient will maintain blood glucose between 70 and 120 mg/dL by eating his 1800-cal ADA diet and taking insulin injections as scheduled.

| Nursing Anxiety Interventions | Patient Responses (Evaluation) |
| --- | --- |
| 1. Assess current level of anxiety | 1. Appeared anxious during hypoglycemic episode |
| 2. Use empathy | 2. Verbalized concerns about disease |
| 3. Use therapeutic touch | 3. Accepted touch, eased anxiety |
| 4. Use therapeutic humor | 4. Responded by smiling, eased anxiety |

*Impressions: Patient stated he was concerned about learning how to give his own injections and how to prepare meals. Therapeutic communication techniques effective in controlling anxiety and establishing open communication.*

■ *Figure* 5-1

**Steps 4 and 5 of the concept map care planning process.**    *(Continued)*

| Problem No. 3 | Deficient Knowledge |
| --- | --- |

**Goal:** Increase knowledge

**Outcome:** Patient decides in collaboration with the nurse what aspects of diabetic teaching protocol he would like to focus on for the day.

| Nursing Education Interventions | Patient Responses (Evaluation) |
| --- | --- |
| 1. Assess current level of knowledge and establish what the patient most wants to learn about during the day of care. | 1. Wants to know about hypoglycemia, Accu-check monitoring, and insulin injections |
| 2. Assess resources available for teaching such as diabetic educator, dietitian, programs, movies, etc. | 2. Diabetes educator visited and will start classes at outpatient clinic when patient discharged |
| 3. See teaching plan:<br>—What diabetes is and how it affects health (signs and symptoms)<br>—Medications<br>—Diet<br>—Skin care<br>—Exercise/activity | 3. Focused on signs and symptoms, use of Accu-check, drawing up insulin<br>See teaching plan for evaluation of learning |

*Impressions: Needs continued practice to use Accu-check. Did not need insulin this shift so could not practice self-administration. Did correctly draw up the medication. Can state the signs of hypoglycemia and hyperglycemia. Review of menus not done due to lack of time.*

| Problem No. 4 | Ineffective Tissue Perfusion (peripheral) |
| --- | --- |

**Goal:** Maintain optimal tissue perfusion and circulation

**Outcome:** Vital signs remain close to normal, no skin breakdown. Patient gets up at least twice, sits in a chair, and does range-of-motion exercises with additional walking with assistance if able.

| Nursing Tissue Perfusion Interventions | Patient Responses (Evaluation) | |
| --- | --- | --- |
| 1. Monitor VS q4h | 1. 0800 BP = 140/85, T = 98, P = 86, R = 20<br>1230 BP = 128/74, T = 98.4, P = 72, R = 18 | |
| 2. Give atenolol, check BP/P before administration | 2. 0900 BP = 148/84, P = 82 | 1330 BP = 124/78, P = 74 |
| 3. Chair x 2 | 3. 0900 for 60 min | 1330 for 60 min |
| 4. ROM extremities q2h if in bed | 4. Does active ROM q2h while in bed and in chair | |
| 5. Walk w/ assistance if able | 5. Ambulated to BR without assistance | |
| 6. Assess skin for ulcers | 6. No redness or broken areas | |

*Impressions: BP controlled with medication, no orthostatic hypotension, strength improving, ambulating well, no skin breakdown*

| Problem No. 5 | Impaired Physical Mobility |
| --- | --- |

**Goal:** Prevent complications of immobility and prevent falls

**Outcome:** Patient ambulates to chair and walks if able, otherwise does range of motion exercises

| Nursing Mobility Interventions | Patient Responses (Evaluation) |
| --- | --- |
| Covered under nutrition and altered tissue perfusion | |

*Impressions: As above.*

| Problem No. 6 | Impaired Urinary Elimination |
| --- | --- |

**Goal:** Maintain normal urinary elimination

**Outcome:** Intake and output approaching normal values, no polyuria

| Nursing Urinary Elimination Interventions | Patient Responses (Evaluation) |
| --- | --- |
| Covered under nutrition | |

*Impressions: No polyuria, output listed above.*

■ *Figure 5-1* (continued)

Steps 4 and 5 of the concept map care planning process.

## Finding Medications

After the assessment and report phase, the next step is to find all your medications for the shift. You already checked the medication administration record and made updates. But now you have to find the drugs. Check to make sure all the pills, injections, liquids, eye drops, inhalants, IV medications, and other required items are on the unit. Medications may be in a medication cart, a refrigerator, or at the bedside. Some may come from a computerized dispenser. Carefully check all currently available drugs. For a drug that is not normally kept on the unit, you may need to follow hospital policy to obtain it. To do so, you may need to call the pharmacy, fax an order, or go to the pharmacy to pick up the drug. Once you have found all your medications, meet your clinical faculty in the medication area to discuss administration early in the shift.

The concept map is particularly useful as you and your clinical faculty analyze relationships between the patient's blood work, physical assessment data, and medications. For example, the discussion of the relationship between insulin, blood glucose level, and appetite is facilitated because all of these items are in the same diagnostic box. Likewise, a discussion of the need to assess the patient's blood pressure before giving the antihypertensive drug valsartan (Diovan) is facilitated because they are in the same box. When you see drugs, laboratory work, and physical assessment data in proximity to each other, the relationships are cemented in your mind. You will soon realize that you must know the blood glucose level to decide whether or not to give the patient his insulin. If his blood glucose level is too low, you could harm the patient by giving the drug.

 ## USING THE CONCEPT MAP TO FACILITATE COMMUNICATION

The concept map care plan is a bridge that facilitates communication between you and faculty. As clinical faculty make bedside rounds, the concept map allows you to easily discuss the patient's progress toward or away from goals and outcomes. As a result of your discussion, you can make notes and revisions on the concept map or problem lists.

## Bedside Communication

Bedside rounds occur periodically throughout the day. Assessment data can be validated or refuted at that time, and maps can be updated as a result of rounds. Faculty comments should appear on your map in a distinct color, such as purple or green, so that these comments are easily visible. Faculty may make written notations instructing you to continue to assess certain aspects of care, to try specific interventions, or to illustrate the finer aspects of the interrelationships of care. Since concept maps show a comprehensive patient picture, they facilitate a thorough discussion between you and your faculty.

For example, the clinical faculty might walk into the room and say: "Let's see your diagram, patient objectives, and intervention lists," and then proceed to ask questions such as: "How is he eating? What's his last blood glucose? Any signs of hypoglycemia? How much is he urinating? How's his blood pressure and pulse? What have you covered so far in your teaching?" These questions can be addressed by review of the updated concept map care plan.

## Reporting Off the Unit

You are responsible for reporting to the patient's assigned staff nurse before going on breaks and before going home. Never leave a unit without giving a report to the patient's assigned staff nurse. Focus the report on the key areas of assessment located centrally on the diagram under the diagnosis. If anything else is abnormal, be sure to tell the staff nurse. Get out your map and use it to remind yourself of what you need to say. For example, as you go to lunch at 11:40 A.M., you tell the staff nurse, "He hasn't had any more signs of hypoglycemia and the 11:30 fingerstick was 100. He did it himself, but still can't remember the exact procedure without help. The doctor wants to be notified about the glucose. The patient's eating in bed right now. Everything else is fine."

 ## IMPLEMENTATION FOR THE DIABETIC PATIENT

The diabetic patient who appeared in earlier chapters will help to illustrate the process of

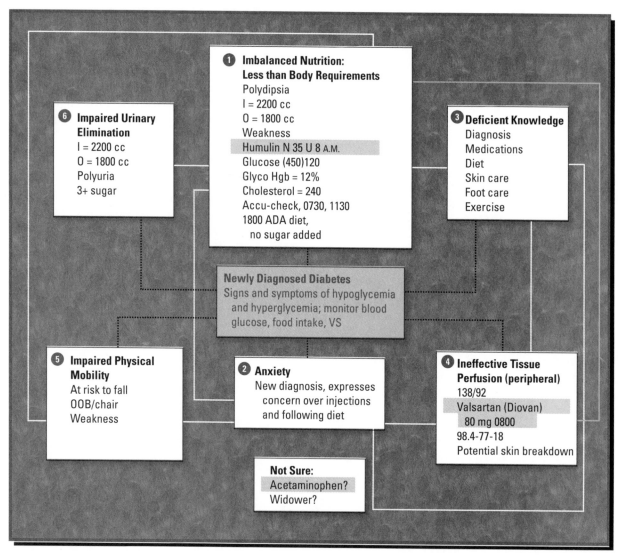

**■ Figure 5–2**

Revised concept map with highlights.
I = intake; O = output.

## Assessment

organizing, implementing, and evaluating patient care. Start by reviewing the concept map shown in Figure 5–2. It has been updated from a review of patient records and the shift report. Medications have been highlighted to make them more prominent.

## Assessment

First, you must do a head-to-toe physical assessment of the patient. Focus on assessing what you

have determined to be essential, which is written in the center box on your concept map under the patient's medical diagnosis. A head-to-toe assessment is the most important way to obtain baseline data at the start of the shift. You must be thorough. If you're checking a patient's lungs, for example, check all lung fields. Student nurses sometimes hesitate to "disturb" a patient to do a complete assessment. The patient may be in pain, he may be immobilized for any number of reasons, or he may simply be asleep. If necessary, get an assistant to hold the patient up while you assess all lung fields and perform the rest of your assessment. Physical assessments are done at least once a shift, more often if the patient's acuity level makes them necessary.

For your diabetic patient, you should ask the patient about signs and symptoms of hypoglycemia and hyperglycemia, obtain results of his blood glucose test, and ask about food intake. As you greet the patient with a handshake, start with a general question, such as, "How are you doing this morning?" Listen carefully to see if the patient says anything that could suggest a problem.

Consider this scenario: He keeps hold of your hand and says that he feels sweaty and light-headed this morning. He is responding to your touch by holding onto you. You ask if he is hungry. He says yes. You ask if he is feeling numb anywhere. He says no. You say, "I'll check your blood sugar and see what it is." You next check his blood glucose level using the Accu-check and find it to be 60. You also find that his blood pressure is 140/85, his pulse is 86, and his respirations are 20. (Quickly write the blood glucose level and vital signs on the care plan so you don't forget them.)

From this data, you conclude that the patient is hypoglycemic but stable. You ask if he can eat his breakfast and he says yes, so you get the tray, open some orange juice for him, and watch while he drinks it. If the tray is not yet available, you can get him orange juice and crackers. Then you immediately report what happened to the patient's staff nurse and your clinical faculty.

Suppose you don't know how to use the Accu-check. In that case, you would quickly take the patient's blood pressure, pulse, and respirations, and conclude from his report that he is probably hypoglycemic but has stable vital signs. Immediately ask your faculty or the patient's staff nurse to check his blood glucose level. Recount the patient's report of symptoms, the blood glucose level, the vital signs, and what you did about the patient's problem. Tell the staff nurse you haven't yet learned to use the Accu-check and ask her to do it. You will have the staff nurse's immediate, undivided attention if you tell her the patient is having a hypoglycemic reaction. This problem needs immediate attention in order for it not to get any worse.

## ■ Establish Mutual Goals

After performing your assessment, you must negotiate with the patient to establish mutual goals, expected outcomes, and a schedule of activities. Use the list of goals, outcomes, and interventions that you already constructed and, in very simple terms, review with the patient what needs to be done. Discuss each of the problems and listen carefully to what the patient believes should be the goals and outcomes of care for the day.

For example, you know that the patient needs to do A.M. care, to get up safely into a chair, to learn about self-care and diabetes, and especially to learn what to do about hypoglycemic reactions. As you review with the patient, use empathy and humor to establish a therapeutic relationship. By using therapeutic communication techniques, you will be better able to find out what's on the patient's mind. For instance, you may find out that he is especially concerned about fluctuations in his blood glucose levels and regulation of insulin with his meals. Of course, you will have things on your mind as well. You will want to discuss his weakness and his risk of falling. Tell him to be cautious when getting up, and explain that you want to be present when he does get up so you can check his blood pressure. List the major items the patient needs to learn for self-care, and let the patient select which aspects of teaching he wants to start with. This portion of the day is about establishing agreements and goals. A successful outcome of your conversation with him thus far would be for him to say that he will not get out of bed without calling you and that he wants to learn how to check his blood glucose after A.M. care. The goals, outcomes, and interventions you established will guide your discussions with the patient in the morning and throughout the day.

## ■ IMPLEMENTING AND EVALUATING CARE

Make sure you do everything you said you were going to do on your plan of care. Some students prefer to check off each item in the list of interventions as they do them so they don't forget to do anything. Your clinical faculty and the patient's staff nurse will be expecting you to either carry out each nursing intervention you listed in

Step 4 or report that it could not get done in a timely manner. For example, say you write that the patient is to do range-of-motion exercises every two hours. You are responsible for checking every two hours and for reminding the patient to do these exercises if he forgets. Failure to carry out all established interventions as planned and in a timely manner is negligent and considered malpractice. Therefore, make sure you keep your faculty informed, no matter how busy they may appear.

As you perform interventions, evaluate the patient's responses to assess his progress toward expected outcomes throughout the day. Record these responses in red ink in the column across from your intervention list (Figure 5–1).

### Completing Step 5—Evaluating Patient Care

Step 5 also includes writing down clinical inferences. Clinical inferences are your impressions about the patient's progress toward the outcomes. You must carefully consider the effective-

ness of your interventions to bring about the expected patient outcomes. If your interventions are not working and the patient is not progressing as anticipated, your clinical faculty and patient's assigned staff nurse are there to help you consider other interventions.

Evaluate the patient's verbal and nonverbal behaviors regarding each item on the intervention list throughout the day. Carefully look for verbal and nonverbal behaviors, plus physical assessment data. Take notes as you go along. You will probably not be doing the interventions in the order you have written them on the intervention "to do" lists, but that is fine. Since interventions are not done in order, you should check off each item as you do it to keep track of what has been done.

### 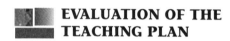 EVALUATION OF THE TEACHING PLAN

In the same way a basic care plan should be evaluated, your teaching plan must be evaluated as

---

**Box 5–3    EVALUATION OF TEACHING PLAN**

**Medications**

- Discussed each medication.
- Patient knew the purpose of each drug.
- Was checking his own blood pressure each week at home using cuff he bought at the drugstore.
- Needs to review side effects and precautions of insulin and valsartan.
- Received printed drug information.

**Environment**

- Patient lives next door to his son, who checks on him daily and will help with meals, medication administration, getting to appointments, and so on.
- Verbalizes activity restrictions in the hospital.

**Treatments**

- Accu-check demonstrated, and patient did his own fingerstick.
- Received printed instructions for operating machine.
- Insulin not given, but patient drew up practice dose without assistance.

**Health Knowledge**

- Verbalizes signs and symptoms of hypoglycemia and hyperglycemia.
- States what to do to avoid hypoglycemia and hyperglycemia.
- Relates symptoms experienced in A.M. to signs and symptoms of hypoglycemia.

**Outpatient Referrals**

- States purpose of doing fingersticks and sequential monitoring.
- Received information for national and regional resources.

**Diet**

- Patient was tired and needed a rest, so unable to finish diet teaching.
- Information given to nurse who will be doing evening care.
- Planning to teach diet with son in attendance.

well. (See Box 4–2 to review the teaching plan in Chapter 4.) While evaluating the teaching plan, focus on teaching methods, responses of the patient or significant other to teaching, and the evaluation of knowledge gained by the patient (Box 5–3). Also note what should be taught and what should be reinforced by the patient's next nurse to ensure continuity of care.

### ▰ Other Outcomes to Review

In addition to evaluating outcomes in individualized concept map care plans and teaching plans, you will also need to evaluate the patient's outcomes against standardized care plans and clinical paths. As you evaluate against the standards, you learn to predict expected patient responses and you can judge how far your patient is away from the expectations for the "typical" patient. Nurses use standardized plans and clinical paths to double-check that everything that was supposed to be done was done. In addition, falls and skin assessments with expected outcomes need to be updated.

 ## INPATIENT VERSUS OUTPATIENT SETTINGS

An obvious difference between inpatient and outpatient units is the acuity level of the patients. Although patients are typically healthier in outpatient settings, you will still need to perform careful assessments, make diagnoses, establish outcomes, carry out interventions, and evaluate patient responses. It is not possible to do an individualized care plan ahead of time for an outpatient. Standardized plans of care and clinical pathways are used as guides for outpatient care. Preparation for an outpatient visit involves reviewing the typical procedures and plans of care that are used in the outpatient setting.

For example, in an endoscopy department, you would review the department's endoscopy procedure flow sheets, preprocedure and postprocedure orders, standardized discharge instructions, and conscious sedation flow sheets. You could use a medical-surgical textbook to review general symptoms and typical diseases diagnosed using endoscopy procedures. You also must be aware of possible complications during

and after the procedure and carefully monitor patients throughout their time in the department.

After reviewing these materials, it would be possible for you to make predictions about possible key diagnoses and develop a concept map that might look something like Figure 5–3.

Once you and the patient arrive on the endoscopy outpatient unit, there is assessment data that must be gathered. For example, Figure 5–4 shows information gathered from a 47-year-old woman before she had an endoscopy procedure in the outpatient department.

During the procedure, the patient's blood pressure, pulses, respirations, pulse oximetry, and level of consciousness will be carefully monitored.

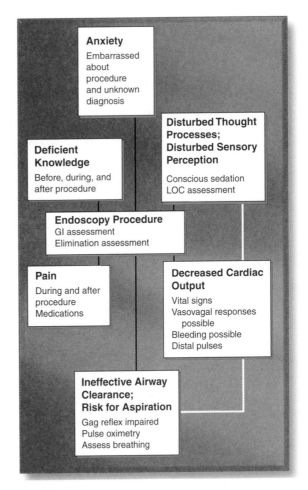

### ▰ *Figure* 5–3

**Endoscopy procedure concept map diagram.**

| | |
|---|---|
| *Reason for procedure* | *Recheck site where large polyp was removed and patient had large blood loss during removal procedure* |
| *Medical diagnosis* | *Polyps* |
| *Procedure* | *Colonoscopy with possible biopsy, polypectomy, or both* |
| *IV* | *No. 18 angiocatheter with 1000 cc 0.9% normal saline solution in right antecubital space* |
| *Vital signs* | *BP = 133/70*<br>*T = 95.8°F*<br>*P = 68*<br>*R = 20* |
| *Height and weight* | *5'5"*<br>*120 lb* |
| *Review of systems* | *WNL all systems*<br>*SaO$_2$ 99%* |
| *Psychosocial-cultural assessment* | *Catholic*<br>*Married*<br>*Anthem insurance*<br>*Manager of a credit union*<br>*During head-to-toe assessment, patient said she was nervous and afraid because of bad experience with bleeding when polyp was removed during the last procedure. Said she wanted to be completely knocked out for the procedure. Wanted a guarantee that she would not bleed like last time. Was visibly shaking.* |

■ *Figure 5–4*

Patient data for endoscopy procedure.

She will receive drugs for sedation and pain. After the procedure, the nurse will perform a head-to-toe assessment with special consideration for the gastrointestinal system and elimination. The nurse will be sure the following outcomes were attained before discharge:

■ Stable vital signs
■ Patent airway
■ Intact gag reflex
■ Minimal nausea, vomiting, and dizziness
■ Oral fluids tolerated
■ Able to ambulate
■ Able to void
■ Comfortable pain level
■ Understands home-going instructions

The pace of care in outpatient settings is very rapid. The nurses rapidly and continually assess, diagnose, plan, implement, and evaluate as the patient responds to the phases of the procedure and recovers from conscious sedation.

## CHAPTER SUMMARY

The focus of this chapter is on organizational strategies to prioritize what must be done during a clinical day. The chapter also focuses on using concept map care plans as clinical organizational tools. Concept map care plans are useful for organizing data in both inpatient and outpatient settings.

Concept maps are used to organize patient assessment information, medications, IV fluids, treatments, and laboratory data when you arrive at the clinical unit. The maps are used to guide your patient assessments and evaluation of patient responses. Concept maps can be used to facilitate communications at the patient's bedside, in the medication area, and when you leave the unit for a break or at the end of the clinical day.

Step 5 of the concept map care planning process is to take notes on patient responses to interventions, evaluate outcomes, and record clinical impressions regarding your patient's progress toward the outcome objectives. You must evaluate the patient's verbal and nonverbal behaviors, assemble physical assessment data, and write notes in the patient response column of the nursing concept map care plan. These notes are the basis of documentation, which will be the focus of Chapter 7.

## LEARNING ACTIVITIES

1. Preconference activity: Students need to make comparisons with other students regarding diagnoses, goals, objectives, and intervention lists. For example, if one student has a postoperative patient with a hip replacement and another student has a patient with a knee replacement, these students should get together and compare plans. The purpose of this exercise is to find similarities common to postoperative orthopedic patients, and to become cognizant of individual differences among patients and treatment plans.

2. Devise, implement, and evaluate a plan of care on a real patient assignment in an inpatient or outpatient setting.

3. Class exercise: The purpose of this exercise is to compare Step 5 patient responses in patients with similar diagnoses. Students should bring a completed concept map care plan to class. Students assigned patients with similar diagnoses should form groups and review patient responses. It should become apparent that, although patients may have similar medical and nursing diagnoses, the verbal and nonverbal responses listed under Step 5 are unique, and progress toward outcomes varies from patient to patient.

4. Compare and contrast the concept map developed for a diabetic inpatient with the concept map developed for an outpatient undergoing endoscopy.

## REFERENCES

1. Standards of Nursing Clinical Practice, ed 2. American Nurses Publishing, American Nurses Foundation/American Nurses Association, Washington, D.C., 1998.

2. Ibid.

# Chapter 6

## Mapping Psychosocial Problems

### OBJECTIVES

1. Identify crucial psychosocial characteristics to assess.
2. Describe how to perform the psychosocial assessment.
3. Integrate psychosocial diagnoses into the concept map care plan.
4. Develop goals, outcomes, and interventions for psychosocial diagnoses.
5. Record psychosocial patient responses.
6. Analyze relationships between psychosocial and physical diagnoses.

The purpose of this chapter is to expand on the assessment, diagnosis, planning, implementation, and evaluation of psychosocial problems. The patient profile database is focused on collection of relevant data the night before clinical (or day of clinical), primarily from patient records and in some cases a brief introduction to the patient and a brief discussion with the patient's staff nurse. Most of the data available from patient records is primarily physical in nature, with only a small amount of psychosocial information. Therefore, you will need to interact with patients directly to adequately assess their psychosocial problems.

You need time to interact with patients to establish therapeutic relationships with them. During patient interactions, you need to learn to use therapeutic communication techniques in identifying psychosocial problems and planning, intervention, and evaluation of patient responses. This chapter will focus on how to develop concept map care plans for psychosocial problems.

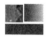 **PSYCHOSOCIAL, CULTURAL, AND DEVELOPMENTAL ASSESSMENT**

Fundamental to the entire care planning and delivery process is your ability to communicate therapeutically and to form a therapeutic relationship. Therapeutic communication is critical to accurate psychosocial, cultural, and developmental assessment. It also forms the foundation of patient teaching. Assessing a patient's psychosocial, cultural, and developmental status is not the same as taking her history and her physical. In contrast to the history and the physical, the psychosocial assessment should not be based on direct questioning or interviewing.

Your objective is to develop rapport with your patients. Nurses must be able to have a comfortable conversation with a patient. The purpose of developing rapport is to help the patient relax enough to verbalize psychosocial concerns whenever they arise. Thus, the psychosocial assessment is integrated into and continues throughout basic patient care. You may have a number of physical goals to attain with your patient, such as improving skin integrity, decreasing pain, increasing tissue perfusion, improving gas exchange, and improving nutrition; you will also need to work simultaneously on assessing the patient's psychosocial problems.

Simultaneous assessment and intervention can be a difficult concept to internalize and perform. But you and your patient are both assessing and responding to each other on a minute-to-minute basis. As a professional nurse, your assessments and responses must be finely tuned to move the patient toward a healthier physical and psychosocial state (or a peaceful death), even while you are in the process of gathering data. You must learn the components of the psychosocial assessment very well so you know what to tune in on. Then, you must learn the appropriate psychosocial responses to the assessment data you gather. Psychosocial guidelines in Box 6–1 and the psychosocial tool that appears in Figure 6–5 have been developed to use during clinical interactions with patients.

The purpose of this assessment tool is to serve as a general critical-thinking guide for assessing psychosocial and cultural problems, and for taking notes. These problems can be very complex, perhaps even more complex than physical problems. There are numerous psychosocial nursing diagnoses, and it helps to have a foundational assessment tool as a general guideline. Therefore, the purpose of this assessment tool is to give you a starting point for collecting psychosocial data. It contains nine important components, including the patient's current emotional state, life experiences, family, growth and development issues, relations with health-care providers, self-concept, culture, and gender. Each section is numbered to correspond with the tool in Figure 6–5.

## 1. Current Emotional State

Assessment of a patient's emotional state must be continuous. You should be consciously aware of the patient's mood by monitoring her verbal and nonverbal behaviors. Is the patient feeling anxious, fearful, sad, hopeless, lonely, out of control? These are very common emotional reactions. Emotions affect a person's ability to concentrate, and they can interrupt the thought processes of the patient or family member. Without the ability to concentrate, it is very difficult for the patient or family to carefully analyze problems or to learn about self-care during a patient education session. Their learning and problem-solving abilities will be impaired. In fact, emotions impair the individual's overall ability to communicate effectively.

One of the most important therapeutic techniques you need to learn and to use is empathy. Empathy involves making it clear to the patient that you have recognized the emotion that the patient expressed. You must correctly interpret the patient's emotional response and then verbally communicate that understanding to the patient. It is important to acknowledge and accept emotions. For example, you can say "I can see that you seem sad." The purpose of empathy is to encourage ventilation by the patient, as well as for you to demonstrate acceptance of the patient's emotions.

## 2. Life Experiences

Use therapeutic communication to assess and talk about changes in patient's social roles as a result of his health alterations. The role alterations

**Box 6-1**   *PSYCHOSOCIAL AND CULTURAL ASSESSMENT GUIDELINES*

### 1. Current Emotional State

Use therapeutic communication to do an emotional assessment and find out the mood of the patient.

### 2. Life Experiences

Use therapeutic communication to talk with your patient about the circumstances surrounding the need for health care and about the patient's perception of the current situation. How has life changed as a result of the problem? How has this problem interfered with the life and the goals that the patient was trying to accomplish?

### 3. Family

How are family members coping with the situation? Are family members supportive? Who is performing the roles of the patient that cannot be done because of the health problem?

### 4. Growth and Development

What are the growth and developmental tasks relevant to age of the patient? How has this health problem interfered with accomplishing growth and developmental tasks?

### 5. Relations with Health-Care Providers

What has the doctor and other members of the health-care team been saying to them? When are they going home (if applicable)? The aim is to determine the patient's current understanding of the problem. In addition, what type of relationship does the patient have with health-care providers? Are they able and willing to follow directions for treatments (compliance)?

### 6. Self-Concept

As you talk with the patient, what inferences can be made regarding self-esteem and body image as a result of the health problems and situation the patient is in? Does the patient appear to have confidence in her ability to care for herself, or does she have doubts and concerns? How accepting is she of the current situation?

### 7. Culture

As you talk with the patient, assess gender and cultural beliefs and practices that are applicable to the current health-care situation. Key areas of assessment include responses to touch, personal space, eye contact, facial expressions, and body language. Determine the dominant family members and which family members have responsibility for health care. In addition, consider nutritional implications, spirituality, and cultural responses to pain.

### 8. Gender

What are the gender speech patterns present in the situation?

---

may be temporary or permanent, but the change will cause concern for patients and significant others. Talk with your patient about the circumstances surrounding how he came to be in the health-care setting and his perception of his current situation. For example, in a hospitalized patient, determine how his or her life has changed as a result of hospitalization; find out who is at home and how everyone in the family is managing while this member is hospitalized. Consider how the problem has interfered with the patient's lifestyle and the goals the patient was trying to accomplish at the time the problem occurred. Also consider the type of work the patient does and the type of leisure activities he enjoys.

### ■ 3. Family and Significant Others

Social support is crucial to successful recovery. Take time to assess the ability of the patient's significant other to cope with the situation and to provide support for the patient. Family and friends commonly feel stress and strain when dealing with the patient's health problem and with the logistics of maintaining their home life and responsibilities.

### ■ 4. Growth and Development

Assess growth and development tasks as appropriate to the patient's age. The stages of growth and development were described by Eric Erickson[1] and included in Chapter 2. Consider how the patient's health problem is interfering with his ability to perform the appropriate growth and development tasks. For example, in young adulthood, tasks involve establishing intimacy and sexual roles, maintaining friendships, growing independent of parents, and establishing a career. Naturally, a lengthy illness can severely disrupt all of these tasks.

## 5. Relations with Health-Care Providers

The nature of a patient's relationship with health-care providers is very important to assess. It is important to know whether the health-care providers and the patient have been able to establish a working relationship and to develop mutual goals. The first consideration is the patient's ability to communicate. Some patients with impaired cognitive functioning—such as those with Alzheimer's disease—probably will not be able to effectively communicate and make rational decisions. Thus, the family will be working closely with the health-care providers to discuss goals and outcomes.

Also, find out whether the patient and family understand the treatment regimen and whether they agree with and support it. Assess whether the patient and family have doubts or concerns about the plan. While providing care, look for evidence of clear or unclear communication between health-care providers and the patient or family. Stay alert to the level of understanding the patient and family have about the plan of care. You may want to ask the patient or a family member a general question such as, "What has the doctor been saying to you about your diabetes?" Or, "What have the nurses been teaching you about your diabetes?" After listening to the patient's answer, you could then follow with a general probing question, such as, "What do you think of all this?" Another good question to use to determine the patient's level of understanding for inpatient settings is, "Do you know when you are going home?" By staying alert and asking prudent questions, you can get a reasonable idea of the patient's and family's understanding of and feelings about the patient's problem.

Compliance is another issue that comes up in relationships between patients and health-care providers. Some patients and families may be "noncompliant" or "nonadherent" with the treatment plan. The goals and outcomes between the health-care provider and patient or family may not be mutual. For example, a patient with a lung condition may refuse to stop smoking. Not all patients are going to be fully "compliant" with all aspects of the plan of care, and they may be mistakenly diagnosed with **Impaired Adjustment.** First, you must determine if the patient understands what is wrong and has been given explanations about how to stop smoking. You must also determine if the patient has the means by which to implement a smoking cessation plan if he decides he wants to do so. Ultimately, it is the patient's decision to agree or not to agree with any aspect of a therapeutic regimen.

Finally, another common relational problem involves turmoil over deciding what to do. The patient and family may have several health-care options from which they need to pick just one. For example, should a grandmother go to a nursing home, or should she move in with one of her children? Should the patient take chemotherapy for cancer or not? Health-care providers commonly guide patients in solving problems, especially as they examine their options. However, it is the patient's and family's right to select the option that best suits them.

## 6. Self-Esteem and Body Image

As you talk with a patient, it is important to assess the patient's self-concept pertaining to self-esteem and body image. Self-esteem is the value that people place on themselves. Because it isn't appropriate to ask, "How is your self-esteem today?" you will need to try to infer it from the patient's body language, tone of voice, and words. As you interact with a patient, you can get clues to a person's lack of self-esteem by paying attention to expressions of feeling worthwhile or useless. People with high self-esteem usually can openly and honestly express what they think and feel. Even though patients have health problems, those with high self-esteem typically believe they are likeable, are capable of handling the challenge of the health problem, and are effective in dealing with problems. According to

Satir,[2] patients with low self-esteem placate, blame, compute, or distract. The placator tries to do whatever someone else says, not because she really wants to, but because she wants the other person to like her and to not be mad at her. The blamer reacts to problems by yelling and giving orders. Beneath this exterior the person believes nobody loves or cares for him. The computer believes that showing emotions is a sign of weakness; this person lives by logic and rationalizations, although he feels very vulnerable on the inside. The distractor uses disruptions to get attention, has difficulty focusing on the issues at hand, and also believes that no one cares about him.

Closely linked to self-esteem is body image. Body image refers to a person's feelings and attitudes toward the physical body. If a person feels good about how he looks, it improves his self-esteem. If he feels bad about how he looks, it worsens his self-esteem. Many illnesses and the aging process alter the structure and functioning of the physical body, and body image disturbances are the result. Scars, deformities, amputations, weight gain or loss, and hair loss are examples of alterations to body image. They may cause patients to be confused about how they perceive themselves. It takes time to integrate and accommodate changes in physical structure and function.

## ▬ Cultural Beliefs and Gender

It is important to assess the patient's cultural beliefs and practices. The influence of gender during communications is also important to assess. Gender differences in communication are partially derived from cultural background, and thus will be assessed with culture. Cultural and gender issues can both affect plans of care. It is important to note that many people are of mixed cultures and that sometimes families have lived in this country for generations. Everyone has beliefs and behaviors that have been passed down, although the origins of the beliefs and behaviors may not be known. Purnell's[3] model will be used as a guide for assessment of cultural beliefs. Tannen's[4] work on gender differences in styles of communication will guide the assessment of gender based communications.

## ▬ 7. Culture

Parnell's model for cultural competence is an excellent tool for cultural assessment. The components of this model that are most relevant to cultural assessments of patients and their families are outlined in Box 6–2 and include heritage, communication, family roles and organization, biocultural ecology, high-risk behaviors, nutrition, pregnancy and childbearing, death rituals, spirituality, health-seeking beliefs and behaviors, the culture of health-care practitioners, and cultural workforce issues.

### HERITAGE

A person's country of origin commonly plays an important role in the development of her ideas and beliefs. For all, except Native Americans, it is especially important to consider why the person, family, or cultural group migrated to this country. Most immigrate in hopes of a better life, but it may help you to know a more specific motivating factor. For example, migration may have resulted from political oppression, religious persecution, lack of job opportunities, or a natural

---

| **Box 6–2** | *COMPONENTS OF PURNELL'S MODEL FOR ASSESSMENT OF CULTURE* |
| --- | --- |

- ■ Heritage
- ■ Communication
- ■ Family roles and organization
- ■ Biocultural ecology
- ■ High-risk behaviors
- ■ Nutrition

- ■ Pregnancy and childbearing
- ■ Death rituals
- ■ Spirituality
- ■ Health-seeking beliefs and behaviors
- ■ Culture of health-care practitioners
- ■ Cultural workforce issues

disaster. Past economic and political experiences directly affect the individual's ideologies. It is important to consider the patient's and family's degree of orientation to their new culture and their familiarity with the health-care system and health-care providers in this country. Except Native Americans, the rest of us have ancestors that immigrated here. Do you know the circumstances surrounding the immigration of your own ancestors?

## COMMUNICATION

Besides considering the influence of language barriers on communication, you should also consider whether the patient feels comfortable sharing his thoughts and feelings. Cultural communication involves the amount of touch that is acceptable, the amount of personal space expected, the amount of eye contact deemed appropriate, the types and meanings of facial expressions used, and the types and meanings of body language displayed. Temporal relationships are important to understand because the expectations regarding punctuality vary among cultures. In addition, there are differing expectations regarding how to properly address people to maintain respect.

## FAMILY ROLES AND ORGANIZATION

It is important to determine the dominant member of the household: the person in the family who is the spokesperson and decision maker. In addition, the nature of the patient's nuclear family, extended family, and living space are important considerations in the plan of care, particularly regarding the level of support the family gives to the member who needs health care. If family members cannot cope with the problem, other arrangements will need to be made.

## BIOCULTURAL ECOLOGY

Cultural groups have specific genetic, physical, and biologic characteristics, such as skin color, bone structure, and metabolism. These characteristics are noted in the general physical screening examinations. Health-care providers need to screen for specific health problems in different cultural groups because some diseases are genetically and environmentally transmitted. For ex-

ample, sickle cell disease, diabetes, and malaria occur with increased prevalence in particular ethnic groups. This information is routinely available on patient records and is part of the basic history screening examination.

## HIGH-RISK BEHAVIORS

These behaviors include the use of tobacco, alcohol, and recreational drugs; participation in high-risk physical activities; and lack of adherence to important health safety practices. Behaviors may vary with the cultural group and must be explored with each patient. Assessment of high-risk behaviors is typically part of the general screening health history.

## NUTRITION

A patient's diet is integral to many health problems and must be a topic of assessment. It is important that you become aware of the basic ingredients of native food dishes and preparation practices to provide culturally competent dietary counseling. Each cultural group has food preferences. The goal of dietary counseling is to select healthy foods from within the culturally preferred choices, and not to require the patient to follow a typical American diet as part of the plan of care. Cultural meaning may be attached to foods that the patient eats or avoids. Food is often associated with cultural rituals.

## PREGNANCY AND CHILDBEARING PRACTICES

Patients' beliefs and practices regarding fertility, birth control, pregnancy, birthing, and postpartum care vary widely based in part upon cultural background. For example, the selection of birth control methods, the roles of men in childbirth, the positions for delivering a baby, and the preferred types of health practitioners (male or female, midwife or obstetrician) commonly differ among people of different cultural groups.

## DEATH RITUALS

It is important to identify culturally specific death rituals and mourning practices. Each culture has its own view of death, dying, and the afterlife. One of the goals of nursing a dying patient is to provide the means for a peaceful death, and that can only be accomplished if you know the person's and family's death rituals. For example, a Catholic patient may want a priest to administer Last Rites, and a Muslim patient may want the bed positioned to face Mecca.

### SPIRITUALITY

It is important to assess the dominant religion of an ethnic group, and to be aware of the patient's and family's use of activities such as prayer or meditation as a source of comfort. Also, you should know how to contact the patient's religious leaders if the patient or family so desires. Keep in mind that spirituality does not always involve a specific religion. Spirituality involves beliefs about the meaning and purposes of life. The patient's and family's spirituality may be a source of emotional strength and sustenance through trying health-care situations.

### HEALTH-SEEKING BELIEFS AND BEHAVIORS

It is important to assess the predominate beliefs influencing a patient's health-care practices. This includes practices regarding care of the sick, as well as health promotion and prevention. Cultures vary in their beliefs about pain, mental and physical handicaps, and chronic illness. It is important to determine who will assume responsibility for care of the sick, and the role of health insurance in the culture. Included in this category are folklore practices that influence health behaviors. For example, blood transfusions or implantation of electrical devices may not be acceptable to a particular cultural group, although these are common medical practices.

### CULTURE OF THE HEALTH-CARE PRACTITIONERS

When the health professional and patient are from different cultures, there may be a lack of trust if either person considers the other to be an outsider. The gender and the age of the health-care provider are also important to consider in providing culturally competent care. And the status given to health-care providers and to the advice they give varies among cultures.

### CULTURAL WORKFORCE ISSUES

As a nurse, you will almost certainly work in a multicultural environment. Both patients and health-care providers come from a variety of cultural backgrounds. The primary factors related to work include language barriers, degree of assimilation, and autonomy issues as health-care providers from different backgrounds work together. For example, difficulties may arise in the workplace from differing values placed on timeliness and punctuality, differences in learning styles, differences in personality styles, and differing levels of assertiveness. As you develop care plans for patients and families, you must learn to be culturally sensitive not only to patients and their families but also to other health-care providers from different cultural backgrounds.

It is impossible to know the beliefs and practices of every culture, but health-care providers intent on providing culturally competent care continue to learn through traveling, reading, and attending events held by local ethnic and cultural organizations, as well as drawing on the expertise of colleagues. Most important, health-care providers need to learn to effectively conduct a cultural assessment and then analyze and solve health-care problems of patients and their family members from the perspective of the patient's cultural group. Culturally competent health-care professionals must be highly proficient in therapeutic communication.

Of special significance is that health-care providers refrain form making judgments about cultural behaviors and practices that they deem strange or "wrong."

There are many ways to attain a mutual goal. Or, to be philosophical, there are many paths to the same destination. Health-care providers must be resourceful and creative and tailor interventions to suit the patient's culture. They must respect differences and appreciate the inherent worth of diverse cultures. The first step in becoming culturally competent is to become aware of your own values, attitudes, and beliefs. The Learning Activities at the end of the chapter are designed to put you in touch with your own ethnic background.

### ■ 8. Gender

Tannen's views on gender differences may help you to assess and respond appropriately to differing styles of speech in male and female patients.

| Table 6-1 | Traditional Gender Differences in Communication | |
|---|---|---|
| **FEMALE** | **MALE** | |
| Rapport talk | Report talk | |
| Less adversative | More adversative | |
| Cooperative overlapper | Talks alone | |
| Listener | Information provider | |
| Personal storytelling | Storytelling of human contests | |
| Uses tag questions | Does not use tag questions | |
| Conversational rituals: | Conversational rituals: | |
| "I'm sorry" | Joking | |
| "Thanks" | Teasing | |
| | Sarcasm | |

Communication patterns are culturally ingrained, although there may be a biologic basis for gender differences in communication as well. Tannen's research suggests that women speak at least in part to promote intimacy and to form communal connections, whereas men are more likely to focus on hierarchy and attainment and demonstration of status in their speech. As a nurse, you must learn to respond to patients based on the speech patterns you discern. General characteristics of male and female speech patterns are listed in Table 6–1. You may need to alter your communication patterns to suit the gender of your patient. For a more detailed discussion of how to accomplish this goal and what nursing implications may arise, read Chapter 2 of Schuster's *Communication: The Key to the Therapeutic Relationship*."[5]

Rapport talk with patients is an essential therapeutic communication skill because it leads to the development of a trusting therapeutic relationship. The purpose of rapport talk is to establish what the patient thinks and feels about the situation through use of empathy. You will also need to know how to give a specific "skip the details" report of facts about the patient to health-care providers and, as appropriate, to patients and family members. Regarding adversity, you must learn to manage conflict with patients and other health-care professionals. If you have trouble dealing with conflict, you need to learn to use diplomacy and tact, yet be able to speak out and be direct about what's wrong and how the problem could be resolved.

Another communication skill that you and all nurses must focus on and master is assertiveness. The assertive person communicates in a direct, honest, and appropriate manner that does not interfere with another person's freedoms and rights. Assertiveness is especially important in the nursing role of advocacy, where you are actively involved in supporting the rights of patients. You must learn to have balance in a conversation, overlapping or not overlapping depending on the patient's style. To be therapeutic, you must learn how to listen carefully as well as to interrupt tactfully when necessary, and then how to provide information as needed. By listening to a patient's stories, you can help to distract him from his problems. In addition, you must examine your use of rituals. Don't overuse such expressions as "I'm sorry" or "Thank you." Also, be careful with your use of humor so that it is not offensive. Teasing, sarcasm, and put-downs are not perceived as funny by many people.

## PSYCHOSOCIAL/CULTURAL IMPLICATIONS FOR TEACHING

Although you will have already prepared teaching materials the night before clinical, as described in Chapter 4, the psychosocial assessment must be integrated into your plan of teaching. Psychosocial characteristics may prompt modifications in the basic teaching plan that you developed before interacting with your patient. Specifically, assess the patient's mood, life experiences, relationships with health-care providers, self-esteem, body image, cultural beliefs, and gender communication patterns.

Before you begin to teach, find out the patient's immediate thoughts and concerns, and deal with emotions first. An emotional assessment is very important before you start teaching to determine if the patient is ready, willing, and able to learn. For example, if the patient is anxious about the results of a test, you may need to decrease anxiety levels before attempting to teach. If the patient is tired, hungry, or in pain, it is best to postpone teaching until these basic needs are met. As you prepare to teach about diet, you need to find out relevant facts, such as whether the patient is Hindu and vegetarian. You have information on general nutrition to promote healing, but the nutrition teaching needs to be altered to encompass a vegetarian diet.

In summary, the psychosocial and cultural assessment tool is to be used as a guide for collecting data. Bring this guide to clinical to assist you in the development of the psychosocial map. The guide entails eight basic categories of characteristics to assess as you work with the patient and family. However, be aware that more in-depth assessment of a particular area may be needed, depending on the situation. A vast amount of literature exists on each of the concepts in the assessment guide. The guide barely scratches the surface of available knowledge, but at least it provides a starting point for data collection.

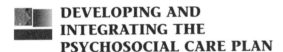

## DEVELOPING AND INTEGRATING THE PSYCHOSOCIAL CARE PLAN

Throughout the clinical day, you will assess, diagnose, plan, implement, and evaluate psychosocial problems. Next, we will develop a clinical case study in detail to illustrate how you can integrate this data into a psychosocial plan of care. A patient with breast cancer and mastectomy will be used to illustrate this process.

Start with the initial patient profile database for the mastectomy patient who was presented in Chapter 3. It is reproduced for you in Figure 6–1. A student nurse collected this data for care of the patient on postoperative day 1. A basic concept map care plan for Steps 1 to 3 could look like what appears in Figure 6–2. Remember that concept maps may vary in appearance, but all the essential data is there.

The concept map summarizes the patient assessment data collected by the student nurse. This map was updated on arrival to the unit for the latest information on the patient as described in Chapter 5. As you can see, the map includes data regarding physical problems, medications, treatments, and laboratory results. Psychosocial problems are present, but not known in detail. The student nurse could infer that the patient may have some form of depression because she is taking the drug Zoloft, and because the removal

of a breast is disfiguring and may influence her most intimate relationships. Therefore, there is evidence to support the nursing diagnoses of body image disturbance and chronic sorrow. As the nurse interacts with the patient during the clinical day, she is able to do a more thorough continuation of the psychosocial assessment and gain more information regarding the cultural and developmental factors that will necessitate modification of the basic plan of care.

After the map has been updated as described in Chapter 5, the student nurse will begin the initial mini-assessment by checking the patient's vital signs, pain levels, and dressing. Confusion would also be a very large safety concern that is a priority assessment. Imagine that as the student nurse goes into the patient's room and says hello, the patient is confused and asks, "Where am I? Where is my son?" She begins to cry and says, "I want to go home." The student nurse may infer that the patient is probably anxious and sad because she is confused and tearful about where she is and who the nurse is. The student may infer that she may also feel very lonely and out of control. The student introduces herself, tells her where she is, takes the patient's hand, gives the patient some tissues, and explains quietly and calmly that she needs to check her blood pressure and dressing and that she is going to take care of her. The student asks if the patient is hurting anywhere and the patient responds, "No, I want my son Bobby." The student nurse tells the patient that she will try to find Bobby, and then she explains that she needs to check with the staff nurse and her faculty and that she'll be back very soon.

After leaving the room, the student nurse's initial impressions were as follows: This patient is anxious. She wants to go home, she's crying, and she misses her son. She also has acute confusion and is oriented only to name. The student nurse adds these impressions to the concept map, as shown in Figure 6–3. Acute confusion was originally included with the diagnosis of risk for injury, but as soon as the student talked to the patient, it was clearly evident that her confusion was a major nursing diagnosis and needed special consideration.

The student nurse then discusses the situation with her faculty, who validates the diagnoses.

# PATIENT PROFILE
## *DATABASE*

## ADMISSION INFORMATION  Student Name ___ *MAB*

| **1** Date of Care: | **2** Patient Initials: | **3** Age: (face sheet) | **3** Growth and Development: | **4** Sex: (face sheet) | **5** Admission Date: (face sheet) |
|---|---|---|---|---|---|
| *12/4* | *AL* | *80* | *Ego integrity vs. despair* | *F* | *12/3* |

**6** Reason for Hospitalization (face sheet):

*Mastectomy*

**7** Medical Diagnoses:(present diagnoses, past diagnoses; physician's History and Physical notes in chart; nursing intake assessment and Kardex)

*Invasive carcinoma in right breast*
*NIDDM*
*Hypertension*
*MI - 1994*

**8** Surgical Procedures(consent forms and Kardex):

*Right modified radical mastectomy*

## **9** ADVANCE DIRECTIVES (NURSE'S ADMISSION ASSESSMENTS):

Living will: ☐ yes ☒ no     Power of attorney: ☐ yes ☒ no     Do not resuscitate (DNR) order (Kardex): ☐ yes ☐ no

## **10** LABORATORY DATA

| Test | Norms | On admission | Current value | Test | Norms | On admission | Current value |
|---|---|---|---|---|---|---|---|
| White blood cells | | *5.6* | *4.8* | Potassium | | *2.8* | *2.8* |
| Differential | | | | Blood glucose | | *230* | *235* |
| Hemoglobin | | *11.2* | *11* | Glycohemoglobin | | | |
| Hematocrit | | *33.2* | *33.1* | Cholesterol | | | |
| Platelets | | *259,000* | | Low-density lipoproteins | | | |
| Prothrombin time | | | | Urine analysis | | | |
| International normalized ratio | | | | | | | |
| Activated partial thromboplastin time | | | | Other abnormal | | | |

## **11** DIAGNOSTIC TESTS

| Chest x-ray: | EKG: | Other abnormal reports: |
|---|---|---|
| Other: | Other: | Other: |

## **12** MEDICATIONS  List medications and times of administration (medication administration record and check the drawer in the carts for spelling):

| Medication/Time of Administration | Medication/Time of Administration | Medication/Time of Administration |
|---|---|---|
| *Heparin 5000 u 10 A.M.* | *KCL (K-Dur) 20 mEq 10 A.M.* | *Ecotrin 1 tablet PO 10 A.M.* |
| *Lasix 40 mg PO 8 A.M.* | *Zoloft 25 mg PO 10 A.M.* | *K-Dur 40 mEq x 1* |
| *Tenormin 25 mg PO 10 A.M.* | *Lanoxin 0.125 mg PO 10 A.M.* | *Darvocet N-100 1 tab, q4h, p.r.n.* |
| | | |
| | | |
| | | |

■ *Figure 6–1*

A surgical patient with a mastectomy: Patient profile database. q.A.M. = every morning; mEq = milliequivalent; PO = by mouth; VS = vital signs; I&O = intake and output.

*(Continued)*

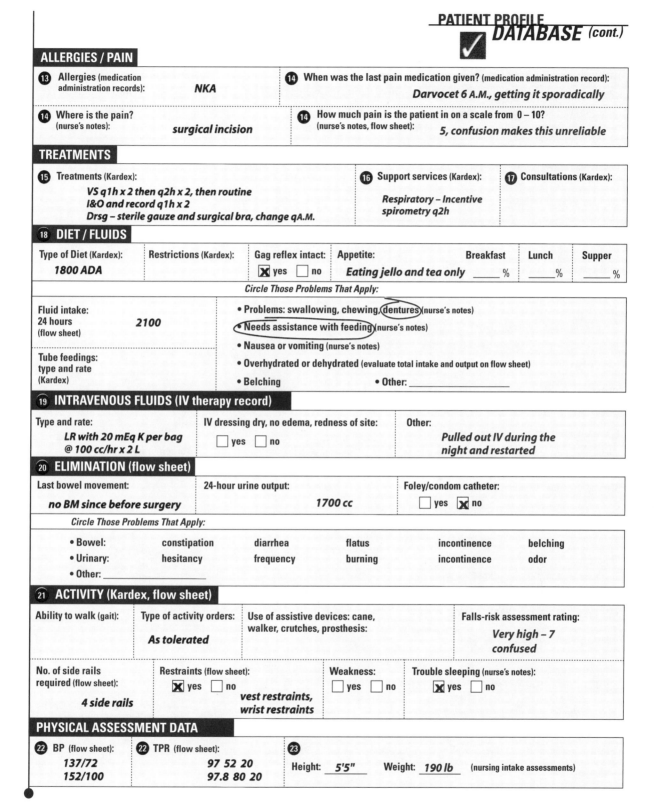

## ALLERGIES / PAIN

**13** Allergies (medication administration records):  **NKA**

**14** When was the last pain medication given? (medication administration record):  **Darvocet 6 A.M., getting it sporadically**

**14** Where is the pain? (nurse's notes):  **surgical incision**

**14** How much pain is the patient in on a scale from 0 – 10? (nurse's notes, flow sheet):  **5, confusion makes this unreliable**

## TREATMENTS

**15** Treatments (Kardex):
**VS q1h x 2 then q2h x 2, then routine**
**I&O and record q1h x 2**
**Drsg – sterile gauze and surgical bra, change qA.M.**

**16** Support services (Kardex):  **Respiratory – Incentive spirometry q2h**

**17** Consultations (Kardex):

## 18 DIET / FLUIDS

| Type of Diet (Kardex): | Restrictions (Kardex): | Gag reflex intact: | Appetite: | Breakfast | Lunch | Supper |
|---|---|---|---|---|---|---|
| **1800 ADA** | | **[X]** yes  [ ] no | **Eating jello and tea only** | ___ % | ___ % | ___ % |

*Circle Those Problems That Apply:*

Fluid intake:
24 hours
(flow sheet)  **2100**

Tube feedings:
type and rate
(Kardex)

- Problems: swallowing, chewing, (dentures) (nurse's notes)
- Needs assistance with feeding (nurse's notes)
- Nausea or vomiting (nurse's notes)
- Overhydrated or dehydrated (evaluate total intake and output on flow sheet)
- Belching  • Other: _____

## 19 INTRAVENOUS FLUIDS (IV therapy record)

Type and rate:
**LR with 20 mEq K per bag @ 100 cc/hr x 2 L**

IV dressing dry, no edema, redness of site:  [ ] yes  [ ] no

Other:
**Pulled out IV during the night and restarted**

## 20 ELIMINATION (flow sheet)

Last bowel movement:
**no BM since before surgery**

24-hour urine output:  **1700 cc**

Foley/condom catheter:  [ ] yes  **[X]** no

*Circle Those Problems That Apply:*

| • Bowel: | constipation | diarrhea | flatus | incontinence | belching |
|---|---|---|---|---|---|
| • Urinary: | hesitancy | frequency | burning | incontinence | odor |

• Other: _____

## 21 ACTIVITY (Kardex, flow sheet)

Ability to walk (gait):

Type of activity orders:  **As tolerated**

Use of assistive devices: cane, walker, crutches, prosthesis:

Falls-risk assessment rating:  **Very high – 7 confused**

No. of side rails required (flow sheet):  **4 side rails**

Restraints (flow sheet):  **[X]** yes  [ ] no  **vest restraints, wrist restraints**

Weakness:  [ ] yes  [ ] no

Trouble sleeping (nurse's notes):  **[X]** yes  [ ] no

## PHYSICAL ASSESSMENT DATA

**22** BP (flow sheet):
**137/72**
**152/100**

**22** TPR (flow sheet):
**97 52 20**
**97.8 80 20**

**23** Height: **5'5"**  Weight: **190 lb**  (nursing intake assessments)

■ *Figure* 6–1

A surgical patient with a mastectomy: Patient profile database. q.A.M. = every morning; mEq = milliequivalent; PO = by mouth; VS = vital signs; I&O = intake and output.

*(Continued)*

**REVIEW OF SYSTEMS**    *Write WNL (within normal limits) if normal and describe abnormalities in space provided: (check nurses' notes and shift assessments for the latest information you can get)*

**PATIENT PROFILE**
**DATABASE** *(cont.)*
☑

**24 NEUROLOGICAL/MENTAL STATUS:** _____

| LOC: alert and oriented to person, place, time (A&O x 3) confused, etc. | Speech: clear, appropriate/inappropriate |
|---|---|
| *confused, oriented to person only, became confused during the evening after surgery* | *Does not know where she is* |

| Motor: ROM x 4 extremities | Sensation: 4 extremities | Pupils: PERRLA | Sensory deficits for vision/hearing/taste/smell |
|---|---|---|---|
| *WNL* | *WNL* | *WNL* | *glasses* |

**25 MUSCULOSKELETAL SYSTEM:** *WNL*

| Bones, joints, muscles (fractures, contractures, arthritis, spinal curvatures, etc.): | Extremity circulation checks (pulses, temperature, sensation, edema): |
|---|---|
| Ted hose/plexi pulses/compression devices: type: | Casts, splint, collar, brace: |

**26 CARDIOVASCULAR SYSTEM:** *WNL*

| Pulses (radial, pedal) (to touch or with Doppler):    3+ | Capillary refill (<3 s): ☒ yes ☐ no | Edema, pitting vs. nonpitting: |
|---|---|---|
| Neck vein (distention): | Sounds: $S_1$, $S_2$, regular, irregular: | Any chest pain: |

**27 RESPIRATORY SYSTEM:** *WNL*

| Depth, rate, rhythm: *20* | Use of accessory muscles: | Cyanosis: | Sputum: color, amount: | Cough: productive, nonproductive: | Breath sounds: clear, rales, wheezes: *slightly decreased in bases* |
|---|---|---|---|---|---|
| Use of oxygen: nasal cannula, mask, trach collar: | Flow rate of oxygen: | Oxygen humidification: ☐ yes ☐ no | Pulse oximeter: _____% oxygen saturation | | Smoking: ☐ yes ☐ no |

**28 GASTROINTESTINAL SYSTEM:** *WNL*

| Abdominal pain, tenderness, guarding; distention, soft, firm: *soft and nondistended* | Bowel sounds x 4 quadrants: *active bowel sounds* | NG tube: describe drainage: |
|---|---|---|
| Ostomy: describe stoma site and stools: | Other: | |

**29 SKIN AND WOUNDS:** _____

| Color, turgor: *skin dry and chapped, poor turgor* | Rash, bruises: | Describe wounds (size, location): *red and edematous, intact, drain sites reddened* | Edges approximated: ☒ yes ☐ no | Type of wound drains: *JP #1 25 cc, JP #2 100 cc* |
|---|---|---|---|---|
| Characteristics of drainage: *both seroanquineous* | Dressings (clean, dry, intact): *clean, dry, intact* | Sutures, staples, steri-strips, other: | Risk for decubitus ulcer assessment rating: *7* | Other: |

**30 EYES, EARS, NOSE, THROAT (EENT):** *WNL*

| Eyes: redness, drainage, edema. ptosis | Ears: drainage | Nose: redness, drainage, edema | Throat: sore |
|---|---|---|---|

### PSYCHOSOCIAL AND CULTURAL ASSESSMENT:

| 31 Religious preference (face sheet): *Catholic* | 32 Marital status (face sheet): *Widowed* | 33 Health-care benefits and insurance (face sheet): *Medicare* | 34 Occupation (face sheet): *Housewife* | 35 Emotional state (nurse's notes): *Anxious, wants to go home, very talkative, does not respond to questions appropriately* |
|---|---|---|---|---|

**Additional information to obtain from clinical units the night before clinical specific to your patient's diagnosis:**

| Standardized falls-risk assessment: ☐ yes ☐ no | Pressure ulcer assessment: ☐ yes ☐ no | Standardized skin assessment: ☐ yes ☐ no | Standardized nursing care plans: ☐ yes ☐ no | Clinical pathways: ☐ yes ☐ no | Patient education materials: ☐ yes ☐ no |
|---|---|---|---|---|---|

■ *Figure 6–1*

**A surgical patient with a mastectomy: Patient profile database.** q.a.m. = every morning; mEq = milliequivalent; PO = by mouth; VS = vital signs; I&O = intake and output.

*(Continued)*

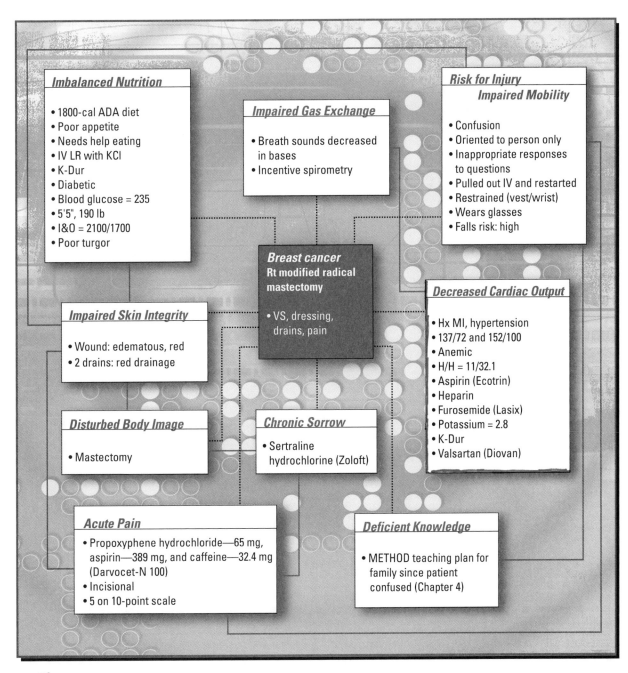

■ *Figure 6–2*
**Concept map: postoperative mastectomy patient. I&O = intake and output.**

Recognizing relationships between psychosocial diagnoses is very important. For example, as anxiety increases, confusion would also probably increase. It is important to recognize that physical problems affect and are interconnected with psy-chosocial problems, and vice versa. Humans respond in a holistic manner to health problems. Lines are drawn in Figure 6–2 and Figure 6–3 to show relationships among the patient's problems.

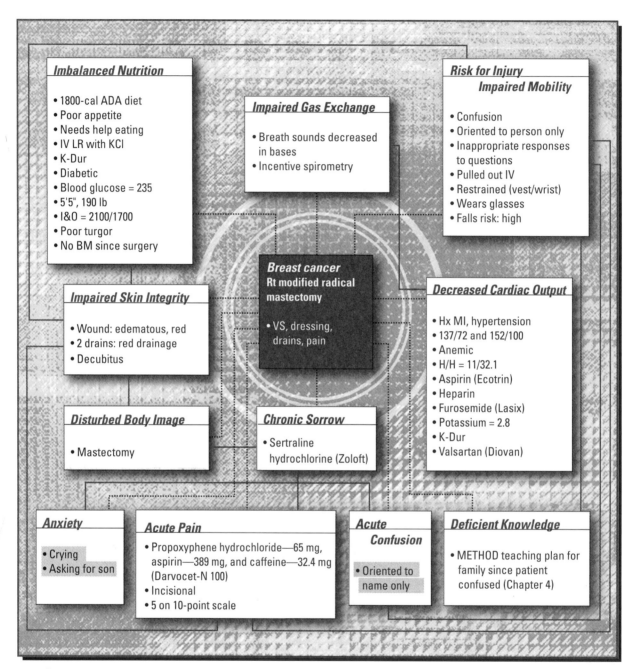

■ *Figure 6–3*

Showing relationships on the concept map. BM = bowel movements; VS = vital signs.

Before writing down outcomes and interventions, you need to take note of how the student nurse intervened immediately when recognized a problem in the above scenario. What therapeutic communication interventions were used by the nurse in the scenario above? Next, plan interventions to help decrease anxiety and confusion. The intervention list has been started for you, along with the goals and outcomes in Figure 6–4. It is important to understand that

**Goal: Decreased Anxiety**
**Behavioral Outcome Objective: Talks about concerns, smiles, rests peacefully**

| Interventions | Patient Responses |
|---|---|
| 1. Use therapeutic comfort touch | 1. |
| 2. Use distraction | 2. |
| 3. | 3. |
| 4. | 4. |
| 5. | 5. |

*Impressions:*

**Goal: Decreased Confusion**
**Behavioral Outcome Objective: No injuries occur, can state where she is and why she is in the hospital.**

| Interventions | Patient Responses |
|---|---|
| 1. Use reality orientation | 1. |
| 2. Use familiar objects | 2. |
| 3. | 3. |
| 4. | 4. |
| 5. | 5. |

*Impressions:*

■ *Figure 6–4*

Step 4 and 5—Psychosocial nursing diagnoses, goals, objectives, interventions, and responses.

psychosocial interventions, primarily communication techniques, are done while continuing the assessment. As you read the continuation of the scenario, identify the therapeutic communication techniques used by the student nurse as she continued the psychosocial assessment along with giving physical care.

The student nurse checks with the staff nurse, who says the patient's son Bobby is coming in soon and that he just called in to check on her.

Bobby states that his mother has not been confused at all at home, and he can't understand why this is happening now. The cover nurse assured Bobby that the doctors were trying to determine the cause for the confusion and that sometimes patients react in such a manner to anesthetics or medications. He also assured Bobby that his mother was being carefully watched. The staff nurse asked Bobby to bring in a family picture or some other object to help reorient his mother.

___◆ **1. *Emotional State***

*What is the patient's mood?*

___◆ **2. *Patient's Life Experience***

*How have previous life experiences affected the patient's perception of the current health problems?*

*How has life changed as a result of the current health problem?*

___◆ **3. *Family***

*What is the patient's and family's perception of the situation?*

*How has family life changed?*

*How are family members coping?*

*Are family members supportive?*

___◆ **4. *Growth and Development***

*What tasks are appropriate?*

*How has this health problem interfered with accomplishing tasks?*

___◆ **5. *Health-Care Providers***

*What is the patient/family current level of understanding?*

*What type of relationship exists with health-care providers?*

___◆ **6. *Self-esteem and Body Image***

*How is the patient's self-esteem threatened by this situation?*

*How is body image changed?*

___◆ **7. *Culture***

*Ethnic background?*

*Which communication factors are relevant and why do you think so? (Touch, personal space, eye contact, facial expressions, body language)*

*Who is the dominant family member?*

*What role does each of the family members play?*

*Who is responsible for care of a sick family member at home?*

___◆ **8. *Gender***

*What were the gender speech behaviors of the patient's son?*

→ ***Note:*** *It is not appropriate to ask the patient direct questions as you would during a history. Information is obtained by observing verbal and nonverbal behaviors and making inferences as you and the patient work toward accomplishing goals and objectives.*

***Figure 6–5***

**Psychosocial cultural assessment tool.**

The student nurse goes back to the patient to finish her assessment and help the patient with breakfast. She makes small talk as she does the physical assessment, using distraction as the therapeutic technique, talking about the patient's pretty blue robe that matches her blue eyes. The patient says that her daughter bought her the robe for her birthday. The patient's son comes in, and she brightens when she sees him and asks him to take her home.

The student nurse continues the psychosocial assessment with the patient's son present, and asks who she lives with. Bobby explains that he and his son live with his mother, who cooks and cleans and takes care of them. He also explains that she is very active with the ladies guild of St. Joseph's Catholic Church. He says that he wants to get her home as soon as possible. He brought in a school picture of his 15-year-old son and puts it on the night stand. The student nurse tells the patient what a handsome grandson she has, and the patient smiles.

The patient's son asks if the doctor had been in yet because he wanted to talk about what was going on and why his mother was confused. The student nurse says she would go out and page the doctor for him. When the student gets back to the room, she says the doctor will be there shortly.

Based on these interactions, use Figure 6–5 to write down a few notes about the psychosocial and cultural characteristics of the patient and her family that have been gathered so far. This is the psychosocial and cultural assessment tool explained in this chapter.

The student nurse next goes over the basic problems and the plans to correct those problems with both the patient and the patient's son. The patient and her son must know the goals and expected outcomes for the day. As the student nurse goes over the plan, she can further assess cultural issues. For example, the student may tell the patient and family that eating foods to promote wound healing is important. She then asks what kinds of foods the patient likes to eat and finds out that the patient prefers the Italian food of her heritage plus sweets of all kinds.

The student nurse discusses the need to keep the patient safe from falls and discusses her activity limitations and the use of restraints for safety. She also discusses the need to monitor vital signs and the care of the wound. In addition, she discusses the need to improve oxygenation and to control pain.

The physician comes in and says that the patient may be reacting to the anesthetic and that her electrolytes are a little off and being corrected. The physician also says that the patient's wound is healing as anticipated. The son explains that he wants to take his mother home as soon as possible and that he and his sister who lives next door would take care of her at home. He believes that once she gets back to her own home she won't be as confused. The doctor says she wants to keep her in the hospital for another day to regulate her electrolytes and to monitor her. The son agrees.

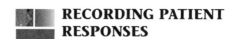

## RECORDING PATIENT RESPONSES

Patient responses to psychosocial and cultural issues should be recorded across from the nursing interventions in the same manner as described for physical interventions in Chapter 5. Remember to look at the patient's verbal and nonverbal behaviors. For example, how does the patient respond to touch? Does she withdraw or smile? Also, write your impressions about the patient's progress toward or away from objectives. Did the patient's responses lead you to conclude that she was talking about her concerns? Was she able to state where she was and why she was there? Record possible patient responses in the Patient Responses column in Figure 6–4.

## CHAPTER SUMMARY

Psychosocial problems are often not known until you have face-to-face interaction with a patient. The focus of the initial concept map care plan is generally on physical information and physical treatments because typically only a small amount of psychosocial information is available in patient records. The bulk of information in patient records concerns physical problems, medications, treatments, and laboratory results.

Assessment of a person's psychosocial and cultural development should be integrated throughout the time you work with the patient. Information collection is more informal than it is during a history and physical, and it should not be done via direct questioning and interviewing. It is accomplished by observing nonverbal behaviors, responses to touch, facial mannerisms, as well as responses to questions.

There are eight major areas to focus on when doing the psychosocial assessment. The current emotional state assessment should be done continually and interventions performed as needed to promote emotional relaxation and comfort. Previous life experiences and how the problem disrupts the patient's lifestyle are important to consider, along with its effects on the family and significant others. Growth and development is disrupted by illness and interferes with a person's ability to accomplish expected tasks of growth and development. Self-esteem and body image can be altered when a health condition affects the patient's feelings of worth and feelings toward the physical body. Cultural assessment involves the consideration of heritage, communication patterns, family roles and organization, biocultural ecology, high-risk behaviors, nutrition, pregnancy and childbearing practices, death rituals, spirituality, and health-seeking behaviors. Gender differences may result in differences in styles of speech.

It is crucial for you to understand the relationship between psychosocial problems and physical problems. Psychosocial problems affect how physical problems are manifested and treated, and vice versa. The concept map serves to illustrate these relationships. You can demonstrate your knowledge of the integration of physical and psychosocial diagnoses by drawing lines to show relationships on concept maps. The goals, outcomes, interventions, and responses involving psychosocial problems are written in the same format as described in previous chapters for physical problems.

Another important point to be made is that both physical and psychosocial assessments are ongoing throughout the clinical day. Changes in goals, outcomes, and interventions sometimes occur on a minute-to-minute basis based on new assessment information or a new evaluation of patient responses. The aim is to provide holistic care.

# LEARNING ACTIVITIES

1. In class, get into groups of three or four and relate examples of therapeutic communication techniques you would use to develop a therapeutic relationship with a patient. For example, empathy is a key therapeutic communication technique. What would you say to show empathy? Other therapeutic communication techniques include supportive touch, humor, problem solving, decision making, increasing patient self-esteem, increasing patient assertiveness, positive reinforcement, encouragement, distraction, reality orientation, reminiscing, anticipatory guidance, and showing positive regard. These techniques were reviewed in Chapter 4. Discuss the patient's specific verbal and nonverbal responses to the techniques. Write them on the board.

2. To get in touch with your own cultural background, do the mini–cultural assessment in Figure 6–6 at the end of this section on yourself. Get together in small groups to compare responses with classmates.

3. In class, get into groups of three or four and relate clinical examples of psychosocial problems that you have encountered in your experiences as nursing students. Give an example to fit each of the categories of the psychosocial, cultural, and developmental assessment guidelines. Give examples of alterations in emotional state, patient's life experiences, family, growth and development, relations with health-care providers, self-esteem, body image, culture, and gender. Elect a spokesperson to share examples with the entire class.

4. Practice developing psychosocial nursing diagnoses answering the following questions:

For each of these feelings, what is the psychosocial nursing diagnosis, and what are the verbal and nonverbal behaviors that indicate each emotion?

*Anxious*

Nursing diagnosis _____

Verbal _____

Nonverbals _____

*Fearful*

Nursing diagnosis _____

Verbal _____

Nonverbals _____

*Sad*

Nursing diagnosis _____

Verbal _____

Nonverbals _____

*Hopeless*

Nursing diagnosis _____

Verbal _____

Nonverbals _____

*Lonely*

Nursing diagnosis _____

Verbal _____

Nonverbals _____

*Out of control*

Nursing diagnosis _____

Verbal _____

Nonverbals _____

For each of the following roles, pretend the role has been disrupted due to a health problem. Write a possible psychosocial nursing diagnosis and a sentence about a situation in which this diagnosis would be appropriate. As a critical-thinking exercise, use a different diagnosis for each role alteration. There are a number of different diagnoses that could be appropriate depending on the situation:

Worker:

Nursing diagnosis _____

Rationale_____

Student:

Nursing diagnosis _____

Rationale_____

Parent:

Nursing diagnosis _____

Rationale_____

Husband/Wife:

Nursing diagnosis _____

Rationale_____

Lover:

Nursing diagnosis _____

Rationale_____

Friend:

Nursing diagnosis _____

Rationale_____

Son/Daughter:

Nursing diagnosis _____

Rationale_____

Sister/Brother:

Nursing diagnosis _____

Rationale_____

Grandparent:

Nursing diagnosis _____

Rationale_____

For each of the following psychosocial problems involving an interaction with the health-care provider, give a psychosocial nursing diagnosis. Write a sentence about why this diagnosis would be appropriate. Since this is a critical-thinking exercise, use a different diagnosis for each situation.

The patient signs himself out of the hospital against medical advice.

Nursing diagnosis _____

Rationale _____

The family cannot decide whether or not to permit the patient to have a feeding tube.

Nursing diagnosis _____

Rationale _____

The family cannot handle all the care required for the ventilator-dependent child at home.

Nursing diagnosis _____

Rationale _____

The cardiac patient states she has no time to do her exercise prescription.

Nursing diagnosis _____

Rationale _____

For each of the situations below involving changes in body image or self-esteem, give a possible psychosocial nursing diagnosis, and write a sentence about why this diagnosis would be appropriate. Use a different diagnosis for each alteration.

The patient refuses to look at the appendectomy scar.

Nursing diagnosis _____

Rationale _____

The patient with a heart attack states, "I'm just no good anymore, I'll never be able to go back to my old job."

Nursing diagnosis _____

Rationale _____

"I'm so ashamed of the way I look without my hair since the chemotherapy."

Nursing diagnosis _____

Rationale _____

"I haven't been outside this apartment for six months because I'm a cripple and I don't want anyone to see me."

Nursing diagnosis _____

Rationale _____

For each of the following examples of cultural nursing care problems, give a possible nursing diagnosis, and write a sentence about why this diagnosis would be appropriate. Use a different diagnosis for each alteration.

The patient says she can't understand how God could have let this happen to her.

Nursing diagnosis _____

Rationale _____

An East Indian woman comes by ambulance into labor and delivery and screams with each contraction. She doesn't understand English, and there is no interpreter available. Her husband is on the way to the hospital.

Nursing diagnosis _____

Rationale _____

The Jehovah's Witness with a hemoglobin of 5 is actively bleeding and is refusing blood.

Nursing diagnosis _____

Rationale _____

5. Practice therapeutic communication techniques by completing the exercise below.

Following are gender communication examples. Specify whether they are typical male or female patterns of communication. Write why you think so and specify what you would say.

The physician comes into the room, says hello, and asks, "What's going on with Mrs. G?"_____

The nurse says to the patient, "It's time to get up to sit in a chair, don't you think so? _____

The patient says to the nurse, "I'm sorry to be such a bother to you." _____

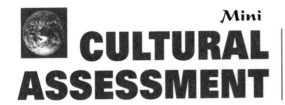

**Mini**

# CULTURAL ASSESSMENT

*Please assess yourself, then we'll exchange views with others from the same and different ethnic backgrounds*

▶ To what cultural/ethnic group do you belong?

------------------------------------------------------------

▶ In what country were you born?

------------------------------------------------------------

▶ In what country were your parents or grandparents (ancestors) born?

------------------------------------------------------------

▶ How closely do you associate with your ethnic group?

------------------------------------------------------------

▶ Whom do you consider your family?

------------------------------------------------------------

------------------------------------------------------------

▶ How important is your family to you?

------------------------------------------------------------

------------------------------------------------------------

▶ In your family, who takes care of infants and children?

------------------------------------------------------------

------------------------------------------------------------

■■ *Figure 6–6*

Mini–cultural assessment. (From:  Schuster, P: Communication: The Key to the Therapeutic Relationship. FA Davis, Philadelphia, 2000, with permission.)

*(Continued)*

▶ In your family, who takes care of sick or elderly?

----------------------------------------------------------------

----------------------------------------------------------------

▶ What do you believe about marriage?

----------------------------------------------------------------

----------------------------------------------------------------

▶ What do you believe about childbearing?

----------------------------------------------------------------

----------------------------------------------------------------

▶ How do you view a nursing mother?

----------------------------------------------------------------

----------------------------------------------------------------

▶ Do you think you should try to control the environment or live in harmony with it?

----------------------------------------------------------------

----------------------------------------------------------------

----------------------------------------------------------------

▶ What is the meaning of life?

----------------------------------------------------------------

----------------------------------------------------------------

■ *Figure 6–6* *(continued)*

► **What do you think about death?**

---------------------------------------------------------------------

---------------------------------------------------------------------

► **How important is punctuality to you?**

---------------------------------------------------------------------

---------------------------------------------------------------------

► **What do you think about the past?**

---------------------------------------------------------------------

---------------------------------------------------------------------

► **What do you think about the present?**

---------------------------------------------------------------------

---------------------------------------------------------------------

► **What do you think about the future?**

---------------------------------------------------------------------

---------------------------------------------------------------------

► **How important to you is moving up in society?**

---------------------------------------------------------------------

---------------------------------------------------------------------

---------------------------------------------------------------------

■ *Figure* **6–6** *(continued)*

▶ **What are the traditional roles of family members in your culture?**

------------------------------------------------

------------------------------------------------

▶ **Who does what tasks in your family?**

------------------------------------------------

------------------------------------------------

▶ **How are decisions made in your family?**

------------------------------------------------

------------------------------------------------

▶ **What place do elderly relatives have in your life?**

------------------------------------------------

------------------------------------------------

▶ **Is the sex of a baby important? Are girl and boy infants treated differently?**

------------------------------------------------

------------------------------------------------

▶ **What rules govern sexual activity for a man? For a woman?**

------------------------------------------------

------------------------------------------------

------------------------------------------------

■ *Figure 6–6* *(continued)*

# REFERENCES

1. Erickson, EH: The Life Cycle Completed. Norton, New York, 1982.
2. Satir, V: The New Peoplemaking. Science and Behavior Books, Mountain View, Calif., 1988.
3. Purnell, LD, and Paulanda, BJ: Transcultural Health Care: A Culturally Competent Approach. FA Davis, Philadelphia, 1998.
4. Tannen, D: You Just Don't Understand: Women and Men in Conversation. Ballantine, New York, 1990.
5. Schuster, PM: Communication: The Key to the Therapeutic Relationship. FA Davis, Philadelphia, 2000.

# Chapter 7

# Concept Maps as the Basis of Documentation

## OBJECTIVES

1. List purposes of documentation.

2. Describe the relationships between the American Nurses Association Standards of Care, American Nurses Association Documentation Standards, and concept map care plans.

3. Specify the basic content of nursing care documentation.

4. Compare documentation formats for standardized forms and narrative progress notes.

5. Identify basic criteria that guide documentation.

6. Use the concept map care plan to identify content for documentation.

*T*he purposes of this chapter are to provide basic information about the process of documentation and to explain the use of concept map care plans as guides for documentation. Documentation, also known as charting, is the legal record of written communication of all patient-care activities. It is crucial that nursing students know how to document accurately and efficiently.

Nurses are legally accountable for following nursing standards of care, and documentation is the written evidence that standards of care were followed. This is also the situation for all other health-care providers involved in patient care. All providers must follow standards of care for their own professional disciplines and provide written evidence that standards were met. Should there be a malpractice claim, charts will be subpoenaed in court, and the legal record will be used as evidence of the health-care services provided and the patient's responses to those services.

Administrators of health-care agencies use patient records to conduct quality assurance audits to monitor the effectiveness and efficiency of all services. Written documentation is needed to ensure quality of patient care by supplying evidence to administrators that health-care providers are doing their jobs. Health administrators are interested in maintaining accreditation from the Joint Commission on Accreditation of Healthcare Organizations (JCAHO). To main-tain accreditation, administrators enforce strict standards of documentation dictated by the JCAHO.

Administrators are also focused on collection of money for services provided from insurance companies, managed care organizations, Medicare, and Medicaid. The amount of reimbursement is based on documentation. Failure to correctly document services provided results in lack of appropriate reimbursement.

Virtually everything that was written on the concept map care plan is documented somewhere in the patient records. Information must be documented concerning all medical and nursing diagnoses that have been identified in the concept map care plan, either through use of flow sheets, progress notes, or care plans. Steps 1, 2, and 3 of concept map care planning, involving development of the concept map itself, will be used as the basis for documentation of assessment data. Step 4, involving outcomes and interventions, will be used to guide documentation of implementation of nursing interventions to attain outcomes. Step 5, notes on the evaluation of patient responses, will be used to guide documentation of patient responses and progress toward outcome objectives. Documentation is a challenge for every health-care provider. Formats for documentation and the exact procedures for documentation are in a constant state of flux. However, the concept maps are very useful tools to help you zero in on the basic content of what must be documented.

## WHAT TO DOCUMENT

The primary objective of the nurse who is documenting care of a patient is to provide evidence that practice standards have been upheld. Assessments, diagnoses, outcomes, interventions, and patient responses must be documented for each encounter with a patient.

It is crucial for nurses to understand the relationships between documentation standards and care standards of the American Nurses Association (ANA) with concept mapping care plans.[1] ANA standards of care are related to documentation standards and the concept map care plan. Carefully identify linkages between practice standards, documentation standards, and concept map care plans as shown in Figure 7–1. Concept maps facilitate documentation because they are cohesive, written, individualized summaries of patient care based on standards of practice.

## WHERE TO DOCUMENT

Everything on the map needs to be documented somewhere. It is initially overwhelming to think that *everything* has to be recorded in medical records. The good news is that not everything has to be personally typed into a computer or written down by your own hand, word by word. Health-care agencies provide nurses with standardized forms to accomplish the daunting task of documentation (Figure 7–2). In addition, succinct written narrative comments are recorded on progress note forms (Figure 7–3).

### Standardized Forms

Standardized forms provide a framework for care. They increase consistency and the completeness of information gathered. They also decrease time spent in documentation. Typical formats of standardized forms include combining checklists and fill-ins with space for a few words. Blank sections are provided on standardized forms to expand on and clarify information to allow individualization of care. As you gain clinical experience at different health-care agencies, you will note many similarities in the contents of standardized forms. Although contents are similar, the layout varies. Each time you switch health-care facilities you need to plan extra time to locate the information needed to develop the patient profile database. You will also be expected to record documentation information on the patient profile database used by the health-care facility.

# ANA STANDARDS OF CARE

### >>> *RELEVANT TO DOCUMENTATION*

> STANDARD

**Assessment:** The nurse collects patient health data.
**Documentation:** Data are documented in a retrievable form.
**Concept map:** Assessment data is collected using the patient profile assessment and the psychosocial tool. Priority assessment data is summarized on the diagram under nursing and medical diagnoses.

> STANDARD

**Diagnosis:** The nurse analyzes the assessment data in determining diagnosis.
**Documentation:** Diagnoses are documented in a manner that facilitates the determination of expected outcomes and plan of care.
**Concept map:** Nursing diagnoses formulated using Steps 1 to 3 of the concept map care planning process are numbered on the diagram to correspond with the outcomes in Step 4.

> STANDARD

**Outcome Identification:** The nurse identifies expected outcomes individualized to the patient.
**Documentation:** Outcomes are documented as measurable goals.
**Concept map:** Individualized outcomes are specific in Step 4.

> STANDARD

**Planning:** The nurse develops a plan of care that prescribes interventions to attain expected outcomes.
**Documentation:** The plan is documented.
**Concept map plan:** Interventions and outcomes are listed in Step 4.

> STANDARD

**Implementation:** The nurse implements the interventions identified in the plan of care.
**Documentation:** Interventions are documented.
**Concept map plan:** Intervention are listed in Step 4 under Goals/Objectives, and as interventions are completed, they are checked off as done.

> STANDARD 6

**Evaluation:** The nurse evaluates the patient's progress toward attainment of outcomes.
**Documentation:** Revisions in diagnosis, outcomes, and the plan of care are documented. The patient's responses to interventions are documented.
**Concept map plan:** Step 5 of the concept map involves the patient's responses to interventions. All revisions written on the concept map are delineated by using ink that is a different color from the initial care plan. Impressions of outcome attainment are summarized.

■ *Figure* 7–1

ANA standards of care relevant to documentation.

## Sample Flow Chart

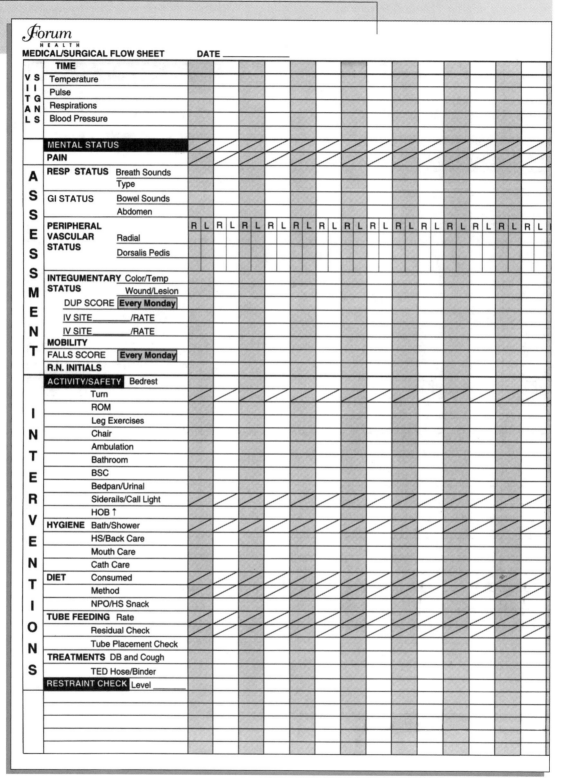

**Figure 7–2**

Sample flow sheet. (From Forum Health, Youngstown, Ohio, with permission.)

*(Continued)*

# Sample Flow Chart
>>> *CONTINUED*

| | | | | | | | | | | | |
|---|---|---|---|---|---|---|---|---|---|---|---|
| | | | **TIME** | | **V** | **S** |
| | | | Temperature | | **I** | **I** |
| | | | Pulse | | **T** | **G** |
| | | | Respirations | | **A** | **N** |
| | | | Blood Pressure | | **L** | **S** |
| | | | MENTAL STATUS | | | |
| | | | PAIN | | | |
| | | | Breath Sounds  RESP STATUS | | **A** |
| | | | Type | | **S** |
| | | | Bowel Sounds  G I STATUS | | **S** |
| | | | Abdomen | | **E** |
| R L R L R L R L R L R L | | | | | **S** |
| | | | Radial  PERIPHERAL VASCULAR STATUS | | **S** |
| | | | Dorsalis Pedis | | **M** |
| | | | Color/Temp  INTEGUMENTARY STATUS | | **E** |
| | | | Wound/Lesion | | **N** |
| | | | DUP SCORE  Every Monday | | **T** |
| | | | IV SITE_____/RATE | | |
| | | | IV SITE_____/RATE | | |
| | | | **MOBILITY** | | |
| | | | FALLS SCORE  Every Monday | | |
| | | | **R.N. INITIALS** | | |
| | | | Bedrest  ACTIVITY/SAFETY | | **I** |
| | | | Turn | | **N** |
| | | | ROM | | **T** |
| | | | Leg Exercises | | **E** |
| | | | Chair | | **R** |
| | | | Ambulation | | **V** |
| | | | Bathroom | | **E** |
| | | | BSC | | **N** |
| | | | Bedpan/Urinal | | **T** |
| | | | Siderails/Call Light | | **I** |
| | | | HOB ↑ | | **O** |
| | | | Bath/Shower  HYGIENE | | **N** |
| | | | HS/Back Care | | **S** |
| | | | Mouth Care | | |
| | | | Cath Care | | |
| | | | Consumed  DIET | | |
| | | | Method | | |
| | | | NPO/HS Snack | | |
| | | | Rate  TUBE FEEDING | | |
| | | | Residual Check | | |
| | | | Tube Placement Check | | |
| | | | DB and Cough  TREATMENTS | | |
| | | | TED Hose/Binder | | |
| | | | RESTRAINT CHECK | | |

## CODES
*\* Needs further explanation*

**Pulse**
AP - Apical pulse
R - Regular
I - Irregular*

**Temperature**
AX - Axillary temp
R - Rectal temp
T - Tympanic

**Mental Status**
A = Alert/0x3
S = Sleeping
O = Other*

**Pain**
0 = None
Scale 1-10*

**Bowel Sounds**
N = Normal
0 = Absent*
↑ = Increased*
↓ = Decreased*

**Pulses**
0 = Absent*
1+ = Weak*
     Thready
2+ = Decreased*
3+ = Normal
4+ = Bounding

**Mobility**
N = Normal
I = Impaired*

**Activity/Hygiene/Turn/Pos**
L = Left Side
R = Right Side
B = Back
P = Prone

S = Self
A = Assist
C = Complete

**Consumed**
G = Good 80-100%
F = Fair  60-80%
P = Poor  60%

**Method**
S = Self
A = Assist
F = Feed

**Resp. Type**
N = Normal
S = Shallow*
D = Deep
L = Labored

**Breath Sounds**
C = Clear
Rh= Rhonchi*
Ra= Rales*
Wz= Wheeze*

**Abdomen**
S = Soft
D = Distended*
F = Firm*

**Skin Temp**
W = Warm/Dry
C = Cool
D = Diaphoretic*

**Skin Color**
N = Normal
C = Cyanotic*
J = Jaundiced*
O = Other*

**Wound/Lesion**
N = None
O = Other*

**Tube Feeding**
C = Continuous
B = Bolus
I = Intermittent

**Level I Restraint Check includes:**
- Visual observation
- Restraint placement
- *Other

**Level II & III Restraint Check includes:**
- Visual observation
- Restraint placement
- Color/temperature check
- Restraint Release for 10 m g2h
- Activity/ROM
- The offer for toileting and nurishment/fluids
- Mental status
- *Other

| Initials | Signature | Shift R.N. |
|---|---|---|
| | | |
| | | |
| | | |
| | | |
| | | |
| | | |

7301005 Rev. 12/97

■ *Figure 7–2* (continued)

135

## Sample Nurse's Notes

$\mathcal{F}$orum
H E A L T H

**NURSES NOTES**
USE "MIDNIGHT LINE" FOR DATING
THE NEW DAY
Date/Time

Addressograph

| HOUR | P.R.N. and Stat Medication | NOTES |
|------|---------------------------|-------|
| 9-8-02 | | |
| 0800 | | Reports pain in surgical incision area "5" on "10" |
| | | point scale, requests pain medication. N Direnzo, I/SU, SN — |
| 0810 | | Given 2 vicodin for pain w/ instruction on use |
| | | of visual imagery exercises & slow deep breathing. |
| | | N Direnzo, I/SU, SN — |
| 0900 | | Reports pain is now "2". N Direnzo, I/SU, SN — |

7301811

■ *Figure 7-3*

Sample nurse's notes.

136

## ASSESSMENT AND REASSESSMENT

### Standardized Assessment/Reassessment Forms

Standardized patient assessments include general history and physical admission assessments, as well as specialized, customized, mini-assessments that occur on an ongoing basis. When assessments are ongoing, they are considered reassessments. You can also think of the reassessments as data for continued evaluation of patient responses. The terminology gets a bit confusing, but after an initial assessment, nurses continue to assess in order to evaluate responses.

As patients enter the inpatient or outpatient health-care system for the first time, there will be a comprehensive history and physical done on admission, with subsequent mini-reassessments customized to the health problems. For example, for a patient with hypertension, after the initial complete history and physical, the focus of subsequent assessments will be on the cardiovascular system. Each area of care such as medical units, surgical units, outpatient clinics, pediatric clinics, and geriatric units will conduct a complete history and physical, and then focus follow-up reassessments/evaluations collecting data specific to the type of service provided.

### Standardized Flow Sheets

Flow sheets are a special type of standardized form used for frequent assessments or reassessments. Nurses always start with a baseline assessment. Subsequent assessments of the same parameter are considered reassessments, but may also be considered evaluation data. As examples, assessment of neurological checks and vital signs are tracked with flow sheets. Flow sheets have formats that allow key data to be seen either in columns or rows and tracked over a period of time. Flow sheets allow easy comparisons to track progress of assessment data over time. A sample flow sheet is shown in Figure 7–2.

### Linking Concept Maps and Standardized Forms for Assessment and Reassessment

The concept map care plan is useful to guide ongoing assessments, reassessments, and evaluation documentation. Make sure you know where to document assessment and reassessment informa-

tion on the agency's standardized forms. Step 5 of the concept map care plan contains information you have written on patient responses, which are reassessments of what was initially assessed using the patient profile database.

## DIAGNOSIS

### Standardized Nursing Diagnoses and Care Plans

The purpose of developing care plans is to communicate goals of care, coordinate patient care, and ensure continuity of care. Historically, health-care agencies and nursing schools have used a care-plan format that has columns for nursing diagnoses: patient outcomes, nursing interventions, rationales for interventions, and evaluation of patient outcomes (see Figure 7–4). In 1992, JCAHO Accreditation standards changed requirements from an individualized plan of nursing care for each patient to recording data about assessments, diagnoses or patient needs, nursing interventions, and patient outcomes (Standard NC 1.3.5) on the patient medical records.[2] Many health-care agencies have subsequently developed standardized care plans for patients with specific diagnoses to decrease paperwork and to meet the ANA and JCAHO standards for practice and documentation.

Nurses need only check, date, and sign appropriate columns in the plan to save time writing about routine outcomes, interventions, rationales, and evaluation of outcomes. Space is usually provided on the standardized forms for individualized outcomes and interventions. A sample standardized care plan from a hospital is shown in Figure 7–5.

Standardized care plans are useful to nurses and student nurses inexperienced in caring for patients with particular diagnoses because expected outcomes and interventions are clearly evident. In each agency you are assigned for clinical experiences, you need to locate and study standardized care plans that may be computerized or preprinted. If care plans are not available, there are numerous up-to-date standardized nursing care plan texts available, as well as medical-surgical texts containing standardized plans of care to guide you in developing the individualized concept map care plan. Experienced nurses have the outcomes, interventions, and

## Sample Column Care Plan

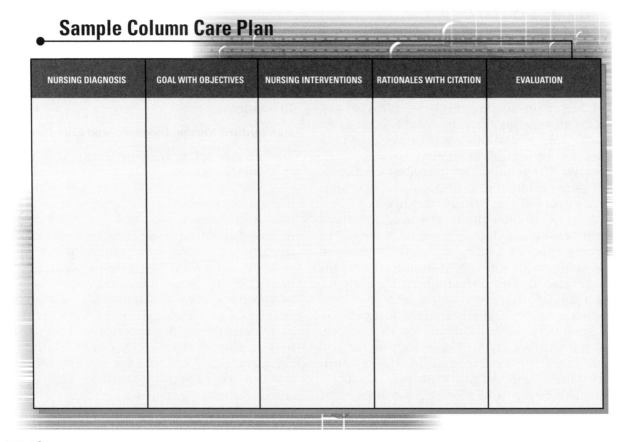

| NURSING DIAGNOSIS | GOAL WITH OBJECTIVES | NURSING INTERVENTIONS | RATIONALES WITH CITATION | EVALUATION |
|---|---|---|---|---|
| | | | | |

■ *Figure 7–4*
Sample column care plan.

rationales ingrained from practice, and have little use for standardized plans of care. There are still numerous complaints from nurses that standardized nursing care plans are just extra paperwork to keep track of.

The current trend in care planning is for agencies to develop and use the standardized interdisciplinary care plans called critical or clinical pathways. These are based on outcomes for specific patient problems such as knee replacements, and are developed by the team of health-care providers involved in the care of a specific patient population.

### Linking Concept Map Care Plans to Standardized Care Plans

Concept map care plans organize and individualize nursing care delivery and increase learning, and should be used in combination with stan-

dardized care plans. At the clinical agencies, use the concept map care plan to individualize the standardized care plans. If there are diagnoses on the diagram that are not included in standardized plans, add them to the standardized plan with appropriate outcomes and interventions.

### Nursing Interventions

#### Standardized Interventions

Standard treatments, medications, and IV fluids are documented on flow sheets. Examples of standard treatments in hospital settings include bath, back care, and oral care. Space is provided on standardized forms for additional treatments to individualize the plan of care. Nursing interventions such as administering medications and IV fluids are very important nursing activities, and they must be carefully documented using

**INITIATED**

Date:

Time:

RN:

**DISCONTINUED**

Date:

Time:

RN:

| INITIATED | | NURSING DIAGNOSIS PATIENT CARE PROBLEM | PATIENT OUTCOMES | EVALUATED | | NURSING INTERVENTIONS | RESOLVED | |
|---|---|---|---|---|---|---|---|---|
| Date | RN | | | Date | RN | | Date | RN |
| | | **1** Body Image Disturbance related to body image change and value in reproductive organ. | Pt will demonstrate adaptive responses related to body image: Pt will ask appropriate questions. State correct information related to procedures and prognosis. State she discussed concerns with partner.<br><br>_____<br>Date | | | **1** Encourage pt's comments and questions about surgery, prognosis.<br><br>**2** Reinforce correct information and provide factual information.<br><br>**3** Encourage verbalization with significant other.<br><br>**4** Discuss hormone replacement therapy.<br><br>**5** Implement pre-op protocol.<br><br>**6** _____<br><br>**7** _____ | | |
| | | **2** Pain related to surgical incision. | Verbalizes minimal discomfort or absence of pain.<br>(ongoing)<br>_____<br>Date<br><br>Progress from IV/IM meds to PO pain meds by second post-op day.<br><br>_____<br>Date | | | **1** Implement acute pain protocol.<br><br>**2** Teach pain rating scale to patient (1–10).<br><br>**3** Reinforce splinting technique if abdominal incision present.<br><br>**4** Assist pt in assuming a position of comfort.<br><br>**5** Keep foley catheter free from pulling.<br><br>**6** _____<br><br>**7** _____ | | |

■ *Figure 7–5*

Sample standardized care plan. (Modified from Forum Health, Youngstown, Ohio, with permission.)

medication and IV administration flow sheets. For example, the antibiotic administered over 3 days is tracked from time to time and day to day across a row of a medication flow sheet. All p.r.n. (as needed) medications will be documented on the flow sheets, and also expanded upon in the narrative notes. Documentation of treatments, medications, and IV therapy is done by listing the dates and times in the appropriate spaces on the flow sheets.

### Linking Concept Map Care Plans to Standard Interventions

Interventions are listed on the front of the diagram under each diagnosis. In addition, interventions are listed in Step 4 of the concept map. All ongoing treatment interventions should be listed on the treatment flow sheet. Medications and IVs are highlighted on the front of the diagram and documented on flow sheets. Specific interventions to alleviate problems will be included with more detailed narrative documentation of specific problems. A sample flow sheet with assessments and treatments is shown in Figure 7–2.

## DOCUMENTATION OF SPECIFIC PROBLEMS: EASY AS "PIE"

Standardized forms for assessment, reassessments/ evaluations, and interventions save a lot of time and organize information. However, there is not enough room on the forms to go into detail for problems. Details of specific problems, interventions, and patient responses are expanded upon using progress notes (also called narrative notes), shown in Figure 7–3.

The content of documentation of specific problems can be easily determined using the concept map diagram of problems as a guide. Each nursing diagnosis must be described in the progress notes. For each nursing diagnosis, documentation can be done in three steps that are as easy as "PIE." First describe the *problem*, second, write *interventions*, and last, *evaluate* patient responses.[3]

### ■ Progress Note P

First, list the nursing diagnosis and then describe the problem by writing abnormal assessment

data that supports the diagnosis. Abnormal assessment/reassessment data is located on the diagram of the concept map under each diagnosis. In addition, assessment/reassessment data is located in Step 5, patient responses/evaluation of the concept map care plan. For example:

> **9/8/01 0800 problem:** Pain (surgical incision) Reports pain in surgical incision area "5" on 10-point scale, requests medication. N. DiRenzo, *YSU, SN*_____

Note that the date and the time are written first, followed by the diagnosis and assessment data. In this example, the data is subjective, because it indicates what the patient reported about pain.

### ■ Progress Note I

Second, describe what was done to alleviate the problem. Write all interventions and instructions given to the patient. The second Note "I" corresponds to the diagram of the concept map where interventions are listed under the diagnoses. In addition, interventions are listed in Step 4 of the concept map care plan.

> **0810:** Given 2 Vicodin for pain w/ instruction on visual imagery exercises. N. DiRenzo, *YSU, SN* _____

### ■ Progress Note E

Third, describe the patient response to what was done. This entails reassessment and evaluation of the initial assessment data. Evaluation of patient responses is listed in Step 5 of the concept map care plan.

> **0900:** Reports pain is now "2". N. DiRenzo, *YSU, SN* _____

In the actual progress notes with explanations deleted, the entry would look like this:

> **9/8/01 0800: problem:** Pain (surgical incision) Reports pain around surgical incision "5" on 10-point scale, requests medication.
>
> **0810:** Given 2 Vicodin for pain w/ instruction on visual imagery. N. DiRenzo, *YSU, SN* _____
>
> **0900:** Reports pain is now "2". N. DiRenzo, *YSU, SN* _____

The preceding example shows the basics of the PIE documentation, but sometimes problems do not resolve quite as easily. In the next example, the initial interventions do not work to alleviate the problem, so more interventions are performed and patient responses are again evaluated (reassessed).

> **9/7/01 0800 problem:**
> Constipation (postoperative decreased GI motility. Reports unable to have BM in 3 days and abdominal discomfort is "3" on a 10-point scale, belching and passing flatus, + bowel sounds 4 quadrants. N. DiRenzo, *YSU, SN* _____
>
> **0810:** Given 30 cc MOM, instructed to drink more water, and given warm tea to drink. N. DiRenzo, *YSU, SN* _____
>
> **1000:** Bowel assessment unchanged from 8 A.M.
> N. DiRenzo, *YSU, SN* _____

Unfortunately, constipation was not alleviated by using milk of magnesia, or by drinking water and tea; additional interventions are therefore needed. It frequently occurs that you will need to continue to work on a problem throughout the day. The nurse has reassessed/evaluated the outcome, and now has to intervene and document additional "I" interventions. There is an ongoing problem, so the evaluation becomes a reassessment and leads directly to the need for additional interventions. This is followed by reassessment/evaluation in the following example:

What was done next?

> **1010:**
> Given Fleet enema. N. DiRenzo, *YSU, SN* _____

## ▬ Progress Note E

Patient response now?

> **1015:** Large brown, formed BM per bedside commode. Patient reports feeling better, Discomfort "0".
> N. DiRenzo, *YSU, SN* _____

This popular documentation system of using standardized forms with progress notes to give details on problems has been termed documentation by exception and also termed a problem-oriented approach.[4] Checklists and fill-ins are useful to quickly record assessments, interven-tions, and evaluations. Problems identified are then expanded on in the progress notes. There is no need to write details about assessments/evaluations that are within normal limits. It is only necessary to write about the exceptions to the norm.

It is very important to be able to provide an in-depth description of the problems with interventions and evaluation of patient responses.

Other mnemonics besides PIE are DAR and SOAPIER. The information contained in the entries is exactly the same. DAR denotes:

- Problem assessment DATA
- Nursing ACTIONS
- Evaluation of RESPONSES

SOAPIER denotes:

- SUBJECTIVE and OBJECTIVE data
- ASSESSMENTS
- PLAN
- INTERVENTIONS
- EVALUATIONS
- REVISIONS

## ▬ HOW TO DOCUMENT: BASIC CRITERIA

Good documentation is concise, accurate, complete, legible, timely, and logically organized. These criteria must be applied each time the nurse makes an entry on a chart.

### ▬ Accuracy of Patient Name, Dates, and Times

Each time something is recorded, the date and time must be included. Check to ensure that the patient's name is on all sheets on which you are recording information. For the same problems, be sure that the dates and times on the flow sheets match the dates and times in the progress notes.

A 24-hour clock, often referred to as military time, is used in most health-care facilities to clearly distinguish A.M. from P.M. hours (Table 7–1).

### ▬ Accuracy of Entries

Always use objective and measurable terms about the patient's behaviors and speech. Objective data includes something you heard, saw, felt, or

| *Table 7-1*  24-Hour Clock | |
| --- | --- |
| 1 P.M. = 1300 | 1 A.M. = 0100 |
| 2 P.M. = 1400 | 2 A.M. = 0200 |
| 3 P.M. = 1500 | 3 A.M. = 0300 |
| 4 P.M. = 1600 | 4 A.M. = 0400 |
| 5 P.M. = 1700 | 5 A.M. = 0500 |
| 6 P.M. = 1800 | 6 A.M. = 0600 |
| 7 P.M. = 1900 | 7 A.M. = 0700 |
| 8 P.M. = 2000 | 8 A.M. = 0800 |
| 9 P.M. = 2100 | 9 A.M. = 0900 |
| 10 P.M. = 2200 | 10 A.M. = 1000 |
| 11 P.M. = 2300 | 11 A.M. = 1100 |
| 12 midnight = 2400 | 12 noon = 1200 |

smelled, termed empirical sensory data. It is strictly factual. It is not appropriate to write opinions, biased statements, or speculations. For example, if you are biased and label the patient a "complainer," you may miss important assessment information. Instead, write a quote about what the patient stated. Write only what you see and let the reader draw any conclusions. Remember, patients have the right to read their charts at any time.

### Legibility

All entries must be legible and in black ink. Write neatly, with correct spelling, and on the lines provided. Ink is used because it cannot be erased and can be photocopied. Illegible writing can lead to life-threatening situations—for example, through medication errors. Always question and clarify illegible writing to avoid patient-care errors. Illegible medication and treatment orders are especially dangerous. In addition, start entries with a capital letter and end with a period.

### Signatures

Always sign the document carefully using the first letter of your name, last name and then title. Traditionally, SN has been the abbreviation for student nurse, LPN for licensed practical nurse, and RN for registered nurse. Since many nursing schools may share the same facility, you will be required to write the abbreviation of your school affiliation along with the title SN, for example N. DiRenzo, YSU, SN.

Never sign anyone else's entry. You are accountable for whatever you sign. The only exception is if a caregiver has left the health-care agency for the day and calls in with information she forgot to document. Then the conversation must be documented in the progress notes, and corrections must be made on the records.

### Correcting Mistakes

When you make a mistake, draw a single line through the words and write the word *error* above the entry, and sign your name or initials. Then make the right entry. Always correct documentation errors promptly, to avoid patient-care errors. Never erase entries, use correction fluid, or scribble out errors. It should not look like data was hidden or tampered with in any way.

### Logical Organization of Information

To ensure correct sequencing of events, document on the standardized forms and progress notes as you go throughout the day. Do not wait till the end of the day to record what happened with patients. It is much easier to accurately remember the sequence of events if recorded shortly after occurrence. Also, do not document in advance. Other health-care providers are dependent on information you document to implement their plans of care, and there is potential for patient-care errors when documentation is not timely or accurate.

Always chart consecutively, line by line, in the progress notes. Never leave blank spaces in progress notes. If you leave blanks, another health-care provider can add incorrect information to the spaces. If space is left after you sign and date an entry, draw a line out to the right margin of the line.

### Writing a Late Entry

Sometimes the nurse may forget to write some data that needs to be included. Start the late entry with the current month, date and time, and then write "Addendum to nurse's note of _____ (month)/_____ (date)/_____ (time)." Never try to squeeze in additional notes near previously written notes. Always make addenda when you forget to enter information. A well-known rule of thumb to guide documentation is: "If you didn't chart it, it wasn't done."

## Completeness

All standardized forms must be filled out completely, with spaces filled in with "not applicable" (NA) if it does not apply to the patient. For example, the menstrual cycle information is not applicable for male patients, and the blank would be filled in with NA.

Overgeneralizations can also be problematic. Specific information is needed. For example, what does "not having a good day" mean exactly? Overgeneralizations waste space, lack objectivity, and are incomplete. The plan of care must be documented on standard forms or using "PIE" on progress notes.

## Omitted Interventions

Sometimes interventions are purposely omitted because of the patient's condition or unavailability of the patient. For example, the patient has a daily laxative scheduled as a routine medication, but now reports loose stools, so the nurse would hold (not give) the medication. The reason the drug was held needs to be included in a progress note, and an order must be obtained from the physician to discontinue the drug. Sometimes the patient may be off the unit when the drugs are supposed to be given, so drugs are not given on time; a note must be made to explain why the drugs were not given at the specified time. Omissions without explanations are considered errors because you must legally do all you were supposed to do or give an explanation as to why it was not done, and then notify the appropriate members of the health-care team.

## Conciseness

Charting entries must be brief, and incomplete sentences are to be used. Eliminate all words that do not change the intended meaning of the entry, including articles such as "a" and "the," and also the subject of the sentence. Use standard abbreviations for conciseness, but only those that are approved by the health-care agency. You can concisely write patient or family comments, but you must put quotes around the actual words the patient spoke. The sample "PIE" documentations previously listed are examples of concise entries. Note that neither the patient's name nor the word "patient" was charted because all entries are about the patient. Also, it is a waste of time and space to repeat in a narrative statement in the progress notes what was covered sufficiently on standardized forms.

## Notes Concerning Other Health-Care Providers

Whether in person or in a phone conversation, document discussions of patient care with other health-care providers. You must record what was discussed and what was done after the conversation. For example:

> **8/8/01 1500** Pain r/t incision: Dr. Morrow notified per phone Percodan did not relieve pain after 1 hour. Pt. states pain is "9" on 10-point scale. N. DiRenzo, *YSU, SN* _____
>
> **1510** Per order, given 50 mg Demoral IM stat. See MAR (medication administration record). N. DiRenzo, *YSU, SN* _____
>
> **1545** Reports pain "4" on 10-point scale. States "much better, but still not gone." N. DiRenzo, *YSU, SN* _____

Never write critical comments about another health-care provider or make entries suggesting an error or unsafe practice. For example, "physician _____ made error in the orders." Instead, write "physician called to clarify _____." Include in the written statement the objective patient behaviors that relate to the error or unsafe practice if applicable.

In the progress notes, always chart changes in the patient's condition, abnormal test results, and the time that the changes were reported to the physician. Additionally, report threats of legal action or bodily harm from the patient or family toward any member of the health-care team or organization. Record and report to the physician and hospital administrators when the patient displays risks to himself, such as drug or alcohol abuse, or if patient is refusing treatment or is unwilling to comply with recommendations. Equipment malfunction is also recorded and reported to supervisors.

# CHAPTER SUMMARY

Concept map care plans are valuable guides for documentation of patient care. Documentation is very important, because it is the legal record of patient care, and in many instances the basis for financial reimbursement by insurance companies, Medicare, and Medicaid. Good documentation is concise, accurate, complete, legible, timely, and logically organized. It is a challenge to learn to do it well, but concept mapping will help to remind you of all that must be documented. As the basis of documentation, you will use the diagram, outcomes and interventions, as well as data collected regarding patient responses to complete standardized forms and narrative notes.

Routine assessments are performed and documented using standardized forms, with specific problems expanded upon in narrative form using progress notes. The mnemonic "PIE" is useful to simplify narrative writing. "P" involves writing about problems, "I" denotes interventions, and "E" denotes evaluation of patient responses. You must meticulously describe the problem, describe what you did about the problem, and then describe the patient response to what you did to alleviate the problem.

# LEARNING ACTIVITIES

1. The following are charting examples taken from actual medical records. For each entry, what needs to be done to correct it?

   ■ By the time he was admitted, his rapid heart had stopped, and he was feeling better.
   ■ Patient has chest pain if she lies on her left side for over a year.
   ■ She has had no rigors or shaking chills, but her husband says she was very hot in bed last night.
   ■ The patient has been depressed since she began seeing me in 1993.
   ■ I have suggested that he loosen his pants before standing, and then, he stands with the help of his wife, they should fall to the floor.
   ■ Healthy appearing decrepit 69 year old male, mentally alert but forgetful.
   ■ Patient has left his white blood cells at another hospital.
   ■ The patient refused an autopsy.
   ■ The patient is tearful and crying constantly. She also appears to be depressed.
   ■ Large brown stool ambulating in the hall.
   ■ Skin: somewhat pale but present.
   ■ Patient has two teenage children but no other abnormalities.
   ■ The patient had waffles for breakfast and anorexia for lunch.
   ■ She slipped on ice and her legs went in separate directions in early December.
   ■ Discharge status: Alive but without permission.
   ■ Patient released to the outpatient department without dressing.
   ■ The patient expired on the floor uneventfully.
   ■ The patient has no past history of suicides.

■ Since she can't get pregnant without her husband, I thought you would like to work her up.
■ The patient will need disposition, and therefore we will get Dr. Smith to dispose of him.

2. Practice writing narrative "PIE" statements for the concept map care plan of the diabetic patient. Use Figure 5–1 from Chapter 5 when the patient had low blood sugar levels.

## REFERENCES

1. Standards of Clinical Nursing Practice, ed 2. American Nurses Publishing, American Nurses Foundation/ American Nurses Association, Washington, D.C., 1998.
2. Accreditation Manual for Hospitals. Joint Commission on Accreditation of Healthcare Organizations, Chicago, 1992.
3. Nursing 99 Charting Tips: Easy as PIE. Nursing 99 29(4): 25, 1999.
4. Eggland, ET, Heinemann, DS: Nursing Documentation, Charting, Recording and Reporting. JB Lippincott, Philadelphia, 1994.

# Chapter 8

## After the Clinical Day Is Over
### Patient Evaluations and Self-Evaluations

### OBJECTIVES

1. Identify standards of nursing performance related to patient care evaluations and performance evaluations.

2. Describe purposes of performance evaluations.

3. Compare formative and summative evaluations.

4. Explain what to do when an error is made.

5. Compare constructive criticism with negative criticism.

6. Analyze criteria for dismissal from clinical.

The clinical day is over and there is very little left to do. The good news is that students spend only about 30 to 60 minutes after leaving the agency evaluating patient progress toward goals and objectives and performing self-evaluations of clinical performance. The time is spent reflecting on clinical performance and patient responses, and writing summaries. The primary focus of this chapter is on professional nursing performance, specifically your performance during the clinical day. The American Nurses Association (ANA) has developed standards of professional nursing performance. The first two of these performance standards include systematic evaluation of the quality and effectiveness of nursing practice and the evaluation of one's own nursing practice.[1]

A very important aspect of a nurse's professional responsibility is a self-evaluation of your performance. Your self-evaluation must be an accurate perception of your abilities. Your clinical faculty will also evaluate your performance weekly with periodic summary evaluations.

In addition to performing a self-evaluation, you will need to finish the evaluation of patient responses and progress toward objectives that you started earlier at the clinical site. You will also need to finish the patient responses to teaching. Students usually need additional time after leaving the clinical site to think about and record patients' physical and emotional behavioral responses. Students also need the time to think about whether the behavioral responses indicate progress toward or away from the objectives that were established for the day of care. Students need to consider the degree to which the patient objectives were attained or not, and write about it under impressions for each nursing diagnosis as described in Chapter 5.

 ## PURPOSE OF PERFORMANCE EVALUATIONS

A performance evaluation is the process of determining how well the nursing student does that which is required. The purpose is not to blame or shame students. The questions to be addressed with the performance evaluation are: (1) "Are you providing safe and effective care?" (2) "What grade did you earn?" and, by the end of the term, (3) "Should you be promoted to the next level?"[2–4]

Your performance will be compared to established standards that define goals to be attained over a period of time. Each course will have expected performance standards that will be stated very clearly and in measurable behaviors. The clinical objectives and specific daily objectives of the course are used as standards to evaluate performance. Performance evaluations are based on standards and objective criteria, not on personalities or whether a faculty member likes a student. Students must own, and accept the consequences of, their mistakes. Sometimes mistakes lead to a bad grade on a test in a theory course; sometimes, mistakes lead to poor patient care or accidental injury to a student. Below are sample objectives for clinical evaluations categorized by nursing process, documentation, and professional qualities.

 ## CLINICAL PERFORMANCE OBJECTIVES

Identify your strengths and weaknesses for each of the following clinical objectives:

## Assessment

1. Prepares each patient profile by gathering complete, relevant information needed to develop a concept map care plan
   a. Defines medical diagnoses
   b. Defines surgical procedures and diagnostic tests
   c. Defines diagnostic test reports
   d. Defines treatments
   e. Defines medications
   f. Obtains health assessment data from the records

## Nursing Diagnoses

1. Develops a concept map
   a. Identifies physiological, psychological, social, cultural, and educational problems
   b. Correctly categorizes data on the map
   c. Correctly prioritizes problems.
   d. Correctly links problems.
   e. Correctly labels problems as nursing diagnoses.

## Planning

1. Develops patient goals, objectives, and nursing interventions
   a. Lists goals and objectives for each diagnosis
   b. Lists nursing interventions to attain objectives
   c. States rationales for interventions

## Implementation

1. Provides safe and effective nursing care
   a. Obtains change of shift information and integrates on map
   b. Checks for updated orders at the beginning of day and throughout the day and integrates on the map
   c. Organizes time, works in an organized manner, and gets care completed on time
   d. Immediately reports assessment abnormalities and problems to the clinical faculty or to a staff nurse
   e. Keeps bed down and locked with side rails up and call light within patient's reach when not with the patient

f. Maintains a safe environment by avoiding activities that could potentially put self or others at risk for injury and by using correct protective actions for patients, coworkers, and self

g. Leaves patient's room neat and clean

h. Continually checks patient safety and comfort needs throughout clinical day

2. Safely and effectively implements all procedures and treatments

   a. Practices and reviews procedures and treatments prior to clinical

   b. Determines basic-care needs and safely performs all procedures without being reminded (examples: C & DB, turning, I&O, ROM, VS, or skin care)

   c. Follows universal precautions with all procedures and treatments

   d. Follows hospital and departmental policies with all procedures and treatments

   e. Displays confidence and composure when carrying out procedures and treatments

   f. Prepares patient/family prior to procedures/treatments

   g. Shows respect for privacy needs

   h. Involves family in care of patient

3. Safely and effectively administers medications

   a. Rechecks the medication records each morning for updates

   b. Questions discrepancies in medication records

   c. Checks for medication allergies on chart and patient arm band

   d. Demonstrates knowledge of medications

   e. Accurately calculates medication doses with 100% accuracy

   f. Accurately calculates IV flow rates

   g. Assesses the Rs prior to administering any medication

   h. Checks appropriate lab work related to medication administration

   i. Evaluates assessment data prior to medication administration

   j. Checks all medications with faculty prior to administration

   k. Uses proper technique when preparing and administering medications

   l. Gives all medications in the allotted time period

4. Safely and effectively teaches and is emotionally supportive to patients and families

   a. Uses the METHOD teaching plan

   b. Provides teaching for patients and family as needed related to METHOD

   c. Demonstrates knowledge of teaching/learning and developmental principles

   d. Answers patient/family's questions and gives explanations in appropriate and understandable terms without causing the patient or family undue anxiety

   e. Provides psychosocial support for patient and families including the use of touch, humor, empathy, anticipatory guidance, relaxation techniques, distraction, reminiscence, and music

5. Communicates effectively

   a. Demonstrates appropriate verbal and nonverbal behaviors in patient/family care

   b. Avoids saying or doing anything that could cause undue anxiety for the patient or family

   c. Reports off to the faculty and appropriate personnel when leaving for breaks or at the end of clinical

   d. Communicates as needed with other healthcare providers in planning and carrying out the plan of care

   e. Informs the faculty and cover nurse immediately regarding any changes in patient's condition or when any problem is encountered

   f. Is pleasant and courteous during all interactions, using therapeutic communication techniques

6. Collaborates with other health-care workers

   a. Actively participates as a health-care team member

   b. Discusses concept map care plan with others (faculty, students, staff)

   c. Assists other patients at the site in addition to those assigned

   d. Interacts effectively with faculty, student, and staff to accomplish objectives

   e. Assists other health team members as time permits

   f. Actively participates in pre- and post-conferences

## Evaluation

1. Evaluates the concept map plan of care
   a. Assesses the patient's progress toward objectives
   b. Assesses patient's behavioral responses to nursing interventions
   c. Modifies the plan of care, as needed, based on evaluation
2. Evaluates self-performance
   a. Objectively assesses self-performance
   b. Immediately admits mistakes and takes actions to correct them
   c. Accepts constructive criticism without making excuses for behaviors
   d. Assumes responsibility for own actions; knows limitations and when to seek guidance
   e. Performs weekly, midterm, and final self-evaluations
   f. Identifies own strengths and weaknesses
   g. Sets own goals and objectives and strives to attain them
   h. Seeks appropriate experiences at agencies to meet individual needs

## Documentation

1. Documents accurately, concisely, completely, and in a timely manner
   a. Records assessment data on appropriate forms (such as flow sheets or progress notes)
   b. Documents without being reminded
   c. Uses PIE format to document abnormal assessment findings and follow-up actions taken
   d. Consults faculty when charting abnormal assessment findings
   e. Demonstrates neatness and organization of charting; uses correct terminology, phraseology, and spelling
   f. Follows agency policy regarding documentation (such as using only approved abbreviations and black ink only) and corrects errors in charting with one line

## Professional Qualities

1. Acts professional at all times
   a. Follows ANA standards of care and standards of nursing performance at all times
   b. Follows all policies of the nursing program regarding clinical conduct
   c. Updates CPR, immunizations, and TB test yearly per nursing department policies
   d. Follows the dress code, presenting with professional attire and behavior during clinical and when obtaining assignments
   e. Submits written work that is neat, organized, complete, and on time
   f. Carefully follows directions
   g. Takes the initiative in arranging for make-up of missed written or clinical work
   h. Is punctual in reporting to or leaving the clinical agency; when ill, calls the agency and faculty prior to scheduled arrival time
2. Acts ethically at all times
   a. Shows respect for patient and family
   b. Calls patient by name and title
   c. Respects patient's personal space
   d. Maintains confidentiality related to patient information
   e. Follows ANA Code of Ethics for Nurses

Your clinical faculty will use critical incidents, rating scales, or both to help you identify your strengths and weaknesses. Critical incident recordings are used to document actual incidents of successful or unsuccessful performance. In using the critical incident approach, you will be asked to list specific actions, reactions, or attributes that were strengths or weaknesses. Two sample critical incident assessment forms are shown in Figures 8–1 and 8–2. You would use the specific behaviors listed above to guide your self-evaluation; your faculty's comments will be right next to yours.

 **CONSTRUCTIVE CRITICISM**

Criticism is a fact of life, and something we all must face. The only way to avoid criticism is to live isolated from other people, but a career in nursing is anything but isolating! We all have had our work, our personalities, and our behaviors criticized at some point. No matter how hard we try, someone is going to be unhappy with us about something; actually, the best any of us can

# SAMPLE 1: WEEKLY CLINICAL PERFORMANCE APPRAISAL

| Student name: | Date: | Week number: |
|---|---|---|

|  | Student comments: | Faculty comments: |
|---|---|---|
| **ASSESSMENT:** | | |
| **DIAGNOSIS:** | | |
| **PLANNING:** | | |
| **IMPLEMENTATION**<br><br>*Procedures/ treatments*<br><br>*Medications*<br><br>*Teaching, guiding, supporting*<br><br>*Communication*<br><br>*Collaboration* | | |
| **EVALUATION:**<br><br>*Patient*<br><br>*Self* | | |
| **DOCUMENTATION:** | | |
| **PROFESSIONAL QUALITIES:** | | |

■ *Figure* 8–1

Weekly clinical performance appraisal.

| Student name: | | Date: | Week number: |
|---|---|---|---|

| Patient's age: | Reason for seeking care: |
|---|---|
| Patient's age: | Reason for seeking care: |

| Meds given: | Skills done: |
|---|---|

| | | |
|---|---|---|
| ASSESSMENT: STRENGTHS/ WEAKNESSES | Student comments: | Faculty comments: |
| PLANNING: STRENGTHS/ WEAKNESSES | Student comments: | Faculty comments: |
| DIAGNOSIS: STRENGTHS/ WEAKNESSES | Student comments: | Faculty comments: |
| IMPLEMENTATION: STRENGTHS/ WEAKNESSES | Student comments: | Faculty comments: |
| PATIENT EVALUATION: STRENGTHS/ WEAKNESSES | Student comments: | Faculty comments: |
| DOCUMENTATION: STRENGTHS/ WEAKNESSES | Student comments: | Faculty comments: |
| PROFESSIONALISM: STRENGTHS/ WEAKNESSES | Student comments: | Faculty comments: |

■ *Figure* 8–2

Weekly evaluation grade sheet. I&O = intake and output; pt = patient.

do is to please some of the people some of the time. Sometimes criticism is utter ungrounded nonsense based on a difference of opinion.[5] In this case, one opinion is as good as any other, provided you believe in respecting others' rights to their opinions. In this situation, be assertive and say, "Your opinion is noted. However, I don't agree and plan to continue _____."

Other times, the criticism received is valuable and helpful, and requires changing behaviors. The valuable and helpful criticism is termed *constructive criticism.* Constructive criticism is based on lack of performance of specific behavioral objectives. Its intent is not to shame or blame on a personal level. Specifically, the intent of constructive criticism from your nursing faculty is to give you feedback on your performance and to help you grow into your role as a professional nurse.

## CARRYING OUT RESPONSIBILITIES AND SHOWING INITIATIVE

As a nursing student, you have many responsibilities that grow with each term in the nursing program. You are expected to perform to the best of your ability and also to take the initiative and look for opportunities to learn new things. For whatever level in nursing you are currently in, there will be specific tasks to perform and specific methods to use in performing them. Once you know your responsibilities, it is up to you to carry them out. If you are unsure of what to do or are afraid of not doing something well, consult with your clinical faculty and get some help. If you don't know how to do something, ask. It is better to admit you don't know something than to have your clinical faculty find out when something is not done. The latter scenario would reflect poorly upon you and—more seriously—would jeopardize care of the patient.

The fastest way to be dismissed from clinical and possibly even from the nursing program is to jeopardize patient safety. Performance appraisals are also used to decide if a student should be dismissed. Not everyone has the ability to be a nurse. Following are some samples of unacceptable clinical behaviors, taken from the Youngstown State

University Department of Nursing Undergraduate Student Handbook:[6]

### DISMISSAL FOR UNACCEPTABLE CLINICAL BEHAVIOR POLICY

**1.** The Department of Nursing reserves the right to dismiss a student whose clinical performance for any nursing course is deemed unsafe as characterized by dangerous, inappropriate, irresponsible, or unethical behavior that actually or potentially places the student, patient, patient's family, or health team members in jeopardy.

**2.** The nursing student must practice within the boundaries of the Nurse Practice Act of the State, the clinical course objectives and guidelines, the Youngtown State University Department of Nursing Policies, and the policies and procedures of the health-care agencies.

**3.** The student's behavior must demonstrate continuity of care through the responsible preparation, implementation, and documentation of the nursing care of patients. In addition, the student's behavior must be respectful of all individuals (patient, patient's family, health team members, and self) according to the AHA Patients' Bill of Rights, the ANA Standards of Care, and the ANA Code for Nurses.

**4.** The student may be suspended or dismissed from the clinical experiences at the discretion of the faculty member.

**Examples of unacceptable clinical behavior include, but are not limited to:**

a. Failure to pick up a clinical assignment or inadequate preparation for clinical experience

b. Attending clinical experiences under the influence of drugs and/or alcohol

c. Refusal to care for an assigned patient based on patient characteristics such as race, culture, religious beliefs, or diagnosis

d. Acts of omission or commission in the care of patients, such as physical abuse; placing the patient in a hazardous position, condition, or circumstance; mental/emotional abuse; and medication errors

e. Disruption of patient care or unit functioning related to poor interpersonal relationships with agency health team members, peers, or faculty

f. Any behavior that affects one or more parameters of safe clinical practice and/or jeopardizes the well-being of patients, patients' families, health team members, peers, or faculty

g. Any behavior that violates professional qualities, such as violation of patient confidentiality or solicitation of patient services leading to personal gain

## CLINICAL EVALUATIONS: FORMATIVE AND SUMMATIVE

Clinical faculty expect that students perform in a state of continuous development throughout the nursing program and that students will make increasing contributions to the clinical care of patients. There are links between performance evaluation, professional growth and development, and the rewards of providing excellent care.[7,9] Faculty and students give feedback to each other in order to evaluate the student's performance, professional growth, and development. The focus is on behaviors and skills. Students and faculty alike receive rewards when the care of patients is done well. Faculty members are very proud of students who receive compliments from both the patients and staff for the good job they are doing or have done, and students are proud of themselves, too. The cycle of performance, evaluation, professional growth, and reward is detailed in Figure 8–3.

### Formative Evaluations

Start out each term by reviewing specific clinical objectives that you will need to meet in order to complete the course. It is very important for you to be aware of what is expected of you. Then, on a weekly formative basis, you and your faculty will jointly select experiences to meet those objectives. For example, during the term just completed, you did not have time to perfect your injection skills, so you ask your faculty to please arrange some additional experiences to develop this skill while still meeting current course objectives.

On a weekly basis, there will be ongoing progress reviews and guidance from your clinical faculty. Students do weekly self-evaluations of strengths and weaknesses with regard to attaining the course objectives. You must objectively write down what you've done well or what needs improvement. Be sure to include any feedback from your faculty in your assessment. Faculty want to see that what they are telling you is registering on a weekly basis. Once you turn in your self-evaluation to the faculty, they will also write their comments. The intent is to monitor behaviors and skills closely, because human lives are at stake. It is very important that you know weekly what your faculty thinks of your performance.

Nurses have awesome responsibilities for the safe care of patients, and you and your faculty are working together very closely to prevent catastrophic mistakes from occurring. Faculty and students alike recognize that mistakes will be made, but avoiding a catastrophic mistake is the prime objective.

### Summative Evaluations

Each clinical course also entails summative evaluations. Usually at midterm and at the end of the term, you and your clinical faculty will have a summative formal conference to review your progress overall toward meeting course objectives. Also, at midterm, individualized performance objectives to accomplish by the end of the term should be established. With weekly formative evaluations, nothing at the summative review should come as a surprise. Your faculty and you will review how you have done relative to the agreed-upon objectives over a period of time. If problems in attaining objectives occur, there must be a discussion about why the objectives have not been met and a new specific plan needs to be developed for meeting the objectives within the time constraints of the term. Specific steps are then decided upon that must be taken for improvement.

Whether the evaluation is formative or summative, there are some basic principles of receiving an evaluation to always remember and do.[9] These include:

## THE CYCLE OF PERFORMANCE, EVALUATION, PROFESSIONAL GROWTH, AND REWARDS

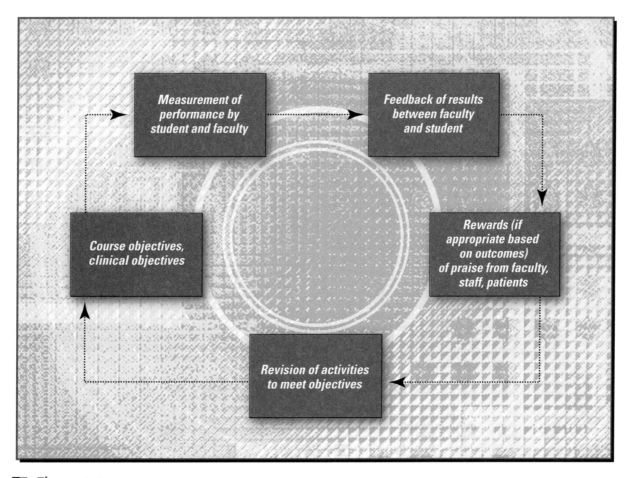

 *Figure* 8–3

The cycle of performance, evaluation, professional growth, and rewards. (Adapted from Mabey, C, et al: Human Resource Management: A Strategic Introduction, ed 2. Blackwell, Malden, Mass., 1998.)

1. View all your constructive criticism feedback as having been given with helpful intent.
2. Listen to your faculty's perspective and avoid excuses.
3. Ask for clarification and ask for examples of the inappropriate behavior.
4. Check with your clinical faculty for mutual understanding.
5. Ask for help and support in the areas of future growth.

## NOW YOU'VE BLOWN IT: MAKING MISTAKES

Say you recapped a contaminated needle, forgot to aspirate, or forgot to wear gloves when doing a subcutaneous injection and there was some bleeding at the site. Now what? First, keep in mind that everyone makes mistakes because no one is perfect. It is part of human nature to make mistakes. You must accept responsibility and be straightforward: "I really blew it by not aspirating." Admit your mistake; do not make excuses because doing so will indicate that you can't accept responsibility for what you've done. Here is a sample excuse from student to faculty: "You made me so nervous by being in the room with me that I forgot to aspirate." Your faculty doesn't want to listen to excuses, and they will lose respect for you if you use them. Blaming your faculty for your lack of performance is certainly an avoidance of responsibility!

Suppose the faculty wasn't there to see the mistake. For example, you neglect to get a patient up for ambulation in the morning because the patient said he was too weak to move. The staff nurse goes to check the patient, asks him if he's walked yet, finds out he hasn't, and irately tells you that patient must be walked immediately. Do you tell your faculty about it or not? Maybe she won't find out and you can cover it up. Honesty and integrity are paramount to safe and effective nursing care. It is much better for

you to tell your faculty about your error in judgment than to let the clinical faculty find out about it from someone else. They want to hear about the error from you directly, because it demonstrates that you take responsibility by owning up to your mistakes. If the faculty thinks that you are purposely covering up an error, it means that you cannot be trusted. A student covering up mistakes is acting unethically because it is dishonest.

Second, don't beat yourself up about mistakes publicly or privately. It is unhealthy to engage in self-recrimination or statements such as, "I'm stupid and will never make a good nurse." A better way to think is this: "I'm intelligent, but I made a mistake that I will never make again." Focus on the behavior that you need to improve. You need to learn and grow from the mistake. Analyze what went wrong, problem-solve, and then don't do it again![10]

## CHAPTER SUMMARY

For successful growth through constructive criticism and evaluation, the aim is to have ongoing exchanges with your clinical faculty about your performance. Both the faculty and the student sometimes need to say hard things in a respectful manner by being open and honest, and trust each other to have each other's best interests in mind. Avoid becoming defensive or argumentative; stick with the facts. Plan on receiving regular, constructive, and candid feedback from your clinical faculty. Your faculty will direct you where to go for assistance as needed (for example, the references to review or the skills laboratory for further practice, the mathematics center, or the writing center).

However, you alone must take responsibility for your own development. You must seek out learning experiences to develop yourself in ways that support the achievement of outstanding nursing care.

## LEARNING ACTIVITIES

1. Compare course objectives from two sequential clinical nursing courses. Describe differences in focus and expectations.
2. Analyze clinical site behavioral objectives for an agency you will use as a clinical site and give examples of behaviors that may be considered strengths and weaknesses.
3. Review your school's dismissal policy and compare it to the sample in the chapter.

# REFERENCES

1. Standards of Clinical Nursing Practice, ed 2. American Nurses Publishing, American Nurses Foundation/American Nurses Association, Washington, D.C., 1998.
2. Clardy, A: Managing Human Resources: Exercise, Experiments, and Applications Workbook. Lawrence Erlbaum Associates, Inc., Mahwah, N.J., 1996.
3. Pynes, JE: Human Resources Management for Public and Nonprofit Organizations. Jossey-Bass Publishers, San Francisco, 1997.
4. Arthur D: Managing Human Resources in Small & Mid-sized Companies, ed 2. American Management Association, New York, 1995.
5. Carlson, R: Don't Sweat the Small Stuff at Work. Hyperion, New York, 1998.
6. Youngstown State University Department of Nursing Undergraduate Student Handbook, Youngstown, Ohio, 2001.
7. Gratton, L, et al: Strategic Human Resource Management. Oxford University Press, New York, 1999.
8. Carr, C: The New Manager's Survival Manual: All the Skills You Need for Success. John Wiley and Sons, New York, 1995.
9. Mabey, C, et al: Human Resource Management: A Strategic Introduction, ed 2. Blackwell, Malden, Mass., 1998.
10. Komisarjevsky, C, and Komisarjevsky, R: Peanut Butter and Jelly Management: Tales From Parenthood, Lessons for Managers. American Management Association, New York, 2000.

# Appendix A

# *Nursing Diagnoses Arranged by Maslow's Hierarchy of Needs*

## Physiological Needs

Activity Intolerance
Activity Intolerance, Risk for
Airway Clearance, Ineffective
Aspiration, Risk for
Breast-feeding, Effective
Breast-feeding, Ineffective
Breast-feeding, Interrupted
Breathing Pattern, Ineffective
Cardiac Output, Decreased
Confusion, Acute
Confusion, Chronic
Constipation
Constipation, Perceived
Constipation, Risk of
Dentition, Impaired
Diarrhea
Environmental Interpretation Syndrome, Impaired
Fatigue
Fluid Volume, Deficient
Fluid Volume, Risk for Deficient
Fluid Volume, Excessive
Fluid Volume, Risk for Imbalance
Gas Exchange, Impaired
Hyperthermia
Hypothermia
Incontinence, Bowel
Incontinence, Functional
Incontinence, Reflex
Incontinence, Risk for Urge
Incontinence, Stress
Incontinence, Total
Incontinence, Urge
Infant Behavior, Disorganized
Infant Behavior, Readiness for Enhanced Organized
Infant Behavior, Risk for Disorganized
Infant Feeding Pattern, Ineffective
Intracranial, Decreased Adaptive Capacity

Memory, Impaired
Mobility, Impaired Bed
Mobility, Impaired Physical
Mobility, Impaired Wheelchair
Nausea
Nutrition, Imbalanced: Less Than Body Requirements
Nutrition, Imbalanced: More Than Body Requirements
Nutrition, Imbalanced: Risk for More Than Body Requirements
Oral Mucous Membranes, Impaired
Pain, Acute
Pain, Chronic
Protection, Ineffective
Self-Care Deficit, Bathing/Hygiene
Self-Care Deficit, Dressing/Grooming
Self-Care Deficit, Feeding
Self-Care Deficit, Toileting
Sensory Perception, Disturbed (Specify) (Visual, Auditory, Kinesthetic, Gustatory, Tactile, Olfactory)
Sexual Dysfunction
Sexuality Pattern, Ineffective
Skin Integrity, Impaired
Skin Integrity, Impaired, Risk for
Sleep Deprivation
Sleep Pattern, Disturbed
Surgical Recovery, Delayed
Swallowing, Impaired
Temperature, Risk for Imbalanced Body
Thermoregulation, Ineffective
Thought Process, Disturbed
Tissue Integrity, Impaired
Tissue Perfusion, Ineffective (Specify) (Renal, Cerebral, Cardiopulmonary, Gastrointestinal, Peripheral)
Transfer Ability, Impaired
Urinary Elimination, Impaired
Urinary Retention

Ventilation, Impaired Spontaneous
Ventilatory Weaning Response, Dysfunctional
Walking, Impaired

## Safety and Security Needs

Communication, Impaired Verbal
Death Anxiety
Disuse Syndrome, Risk for
Dysreflexia
Dysreflexia, Risk for Autonomic
Falls, Risk for
Fear
Grieving, Anticipatory
Grieving, Dysfunctional
Growth, Risk for Disproportional
Health Maintenance, Ineffective
Home Maintenance Management, Impaired
Infection, Risk for
Injury, Risk for
Knowledge, Deficient
Latex Allergy
Latex Allergy, Risk for
Perioperative Positioning Injury, Risk for
Peripheral Neurovascular Dysfunction, Risk for
Poisoning, Risk for
Sorrow, Chronic
Suffocation, Risk for
Therapeutic Regimen: Community, Ineffective
    Management of
Therapeutic Regimen: Families, Ineffective
    Management of
Therapeutic Regimen: Families, Ineffective
    Management of
Therapeutic Regimen: Individual, Ineffective
    Management of
Trauma, Risk for
Unilateral Neglect
Wandering

## Love and Belonging Needs

Adult Failure to Thrive
Anxiety
Caregiver Role Strain
Caregiver Role Strain, Risk for
Family Coping: Compromised, Ineffective
Family Coping: Disabling, Ineffective
Family Coping: Readiness for Enhanced
Family Processes, Interrupted
Loneliness, Risk for
Parent/Infant/Child Attachment, Risk for
    Impaired

Parental Role Conflict
Parenting Deficient
Parenting, Deficient, Risk for
Relocation Stress Syndrome
Social Interaction, Impaired
Social Isolation

## Self-Esteem

Adjustment, Impaired
Alcoholism, Altered Family Process
Body Image Disturbance
Community Coping, Ineffective
Community Coping, Readiness for Enhanced
Coping, Defensive
Coping, Ineffective Individual
Decisional Conflict
Denial, Ineffective
Diversional Activity Deficit
Hopelessness
Noncompliance
Identity, Disturbed
Post-Trauma Syndrome
Post-Trauma Syndrome, Risk for
Powerlessness
Powerlessness, Risk for
Rape-Trauma Syndrome
Rape-Trauma Syndrome: Compound Reaction
Rape-Trauma Syndrome: Silent Reaction
Relocation Stress Syndrome: Risk for
Role Performance, Ineffective
Self-Esteem, Chronic Low
Self-Esteem, Situational Low
Self-Esteem: Situation Low (Risk for)
Self-Esteem Disturbance
Self-Mutilation
Self-Mutilation, Risk for
Suicide, Risk for
Violence: Self-Directed or Directed at Others,
    Risk for

## Self-Actualization Needs

Effective Management of Therapeutic Regimen:
    Individual
Energy Field Disturbance
Growth and Development, Delayed
Delayed Development, Risk for
Health-Seeking Behaviors
Spiritual Well-Being, Readiness for Enhanced
Spiritual Distress
Spiritual Distress, Risk for

# Appendix B

## Nursing Diagnoses Arranged by Gordon's Functional Health Patterns*

### Health-Perception—Health-Management

Health-Seeking Behaviors (Specify)
Ineffective Health Maintenance
Ineffective Management of Therapeutic Regimen
Disturbed Energy Field
Effective Management of Therapeutic Regimen:
  Individuals
Ineffective, Management of Therapeutic
  Regimen: Families
Ineffective Management of Therapeutic
  Regimen: Community
Latex Allergy
Noncompliance (Specify)
Risk for Infection
Risk for Injury
Risk for Latex Allergy
Risk for Trauma
Risk for Perioperative Positioning Injury
Risk for Poisoning
Risk for Suffocation
Altered Protection

### Nutritional-Metabolic

Impaired Dentition
Imbalanced Nutrition: More Than Body
  Requirements
Imbalanced Nutrition: Risk for More Than Body
  Requirements
Imbalanced Nutrition: Less Than Body
  Requirements
Ineffective Breastfeeding
Interrupted Breastfeeding
Effective Breastfeeding
Ineffective Infant Feeding Pattern
Impaired Swallowing
Nausea
Risk for Aspiration

Impaired Oral Mucous Membranes
Deficient Fluid Volume
Risk for Deficient Fluid Volume
Excessive Fluid Volume
Risk for Impaired Skin Integrity
Impaired Skin Integrity
Impaired Tissue Integrity
Risk for Imbalanced Body Temperature
Ineffective Thermoregulation
Hyperthermia
Hypothermia

### Elimination

Constipation
Constipation, Risk for
Diarrhea
Bowel Incontinence
Functional Incontinence
Impaired Urinary Elimination
Perceived Constipation
Reflex Incontinence
Stress Incontinence
Urge Incontinence
Urge Incontinence, Risk for
Total Incontinence
Urinary Retention

### Activity-Exercise

Activity Intolerance
Risk for Activity Intolerance
Adult Failure to Thrive
Delayed Surgical Recovery
Fatigue
Impaired Bed Mobility
Impaired Physical Mobility
Impaired Transfer Ability
Impaired Walking
Impaired Wheelchair Mobility
Risk for Disuse Syndrome
Self-Care Deficit: Bathing/Hygiene
Self-Care Deficit: Dressing/Grooming

*Modified from Gordon M: *Manual of nursing diagnosis,*
1997-1998, St. Louis, 1997, Mosby.

Self-Care Deficit: Feeding
Self-Care Deficit: Toileting
Diversional Activity Deficit
Impaired Home Maintenance Management
Dysfunctional Ventilatory Weaning Response
Inability to Sustain Spontaneous Ventilation
Ineffective Airway Clearance
Ineffective Breathing Pattern
Impaired Gas Exchange
Decreased Cardiac Output
Ineffective Tissue Perfusion (Specify Type)
Dysreflexia
Dysreflexia, Risk for Autonomic
Disorganized Infant Behavior
Risk for Disorganized Infant Behavior
Readiness for Enhanced Organized Infant
   Behavior
Risk for Peripheral Neurovascular Dysfunction
Delayed Growth and Development
Risk for Altered Growth
Risk for Delayed Development
Wandering, Risk for Falls

## Sleep-Rest

Sleep Deprivation
Sleep Pattern Disturbed

## Cognitive-Perceptual Brain

Pain
Chronic Pain
Disturbed Sensory Perception (Specify)
Unilateral Neglect
Deficient Knowledge (Specify)
Disturbed Thought Processes
Acute Confusion
Chronic Confusion
Impaired Environmental Interpretation Syndrome
Impaired Memory
Decisional Conflict (Specify)
Decreased Adaptive Capacity: Intracranial

## Self-Perception—Self-Concept

Anxiety
Body Image Disturbance
Chronic Low Self-Esteem
Death Anxiety
Fear
Hopelessness
Personal Identity Disturbance
Powerlessness
Risk for Powerlessness
Risk for Loneliness

Self-Mutilation
Risk for Self-Mutilation
Self-Esteem Disturbance
Risk for Relocation Syndrome
Situational Low Self-Esteem
Risk for Suicide

## Role-Relationship Family

Anticipatory Grieving
Dysfunctional Grieving
Chronic Sorrow
Ineffective Role Performance
Social Isolation or Social Rejection
Social Isolation
Impaired Social Interaction
Relocation Stress Syndrome
Interrupted Family Processes
Interrupted Family Processes: Alcoholism
Deficient Parenting
Risk for Deficient Parenting
Parental Role Conflict
Risk for Altered Parent-Infant/Child Attachment
Caregiver Role Strain
Risk for Caregiver Role Strain
Impaired Verbal Communication
Risk for Violence: Self-Directed or Directed at
   Others

## Sexuality-Reproductive

Ineffective Sexuality Patterns
Sexual Dysfunction
Rape-Trauma Syndrome
Rape-Trauma Syndrome: Compound Reaction
Rape-Trauma Syndrome: Silent Reaction

## Coping—Stress-Tolerance

Ineffective Individual Coping
Defensive Coping
Ineffective Denial
Impaired Adjustment
Post-Trauma Response
Family Coping: Readiness for Enhanced
Ineffective Family Coping: Compromised
Ineffective Family Coping: Disabling
Ineffective Community Coping
Readiness for Enhanced Community Coping

## Value-Belief

Readiness for Enhanced Spiritual Well-Being
Spiritual Distress (Distress of Human Spirit)
Spiritual Distress, Risk for

# Appendix C

## Nursing Diagnoses

### (Through 14th NANDA Conference)†

‡Activity Intolerance
  Insufficient energy for daily activities
Activity Intolerance, Risk for
‡Adjustment, Impaired
  Inability to modify lifestyle/behavior
‡Airway Clearance, Ineffective
  Inability to clear secretions
Allergy Response, Latex
Allergy Response, Risk for Latex
Anxiety
‡Anxiety, Death
  Uneasy feeling of apprehension and an
  autonomic response, but the source of the
  apprehension is unknown
Aspiration, Risk for
Attachment, Risk for Impaired
  Parent/Infant/Child
Body Image, Disturbed
‡Body Temperature, Risk for Imbalanced
  Hypothermia, hyperthermia, or ineffective
  thermoregulation (fluctuation between
  hypothermia and hyperthermia)
Bowel Incontinence
Breastfeeding, Effective
Breastfeeding, Ineffective
Breastfeeding, Interrupted
‡Breathing Pattern, Ineffective
  Inspiration/expiration is not adequate
‡Cardiac Output, Decreased
  Inadequate cardiac output
Caregiver Role Strain
Caregiver Role Strain, Risk for
Communication, Impaired Verbal
‡Conflict, Decisional
  State of uncertainty about a course of
  action
Conflict, Parental Role
Confusion, Acute
Confusion, Chronic

Constipation
‡Constipation, Perceived
  The patient believes that he or she is
  constipated and abuses laxatives, enemas,
  and suppositories to ensure a daily bowel
  movement
Constipation, Risk for
‡Coping, Ineffective
  Inability to appraise stressors or to use
  available stressors
‡Coping, Ineffective Community
  Community activities are unsatisfactory for
  meeting needs of the community
‡Coping, Readiness for Enhanced Community
    Coping
  Community activities to facilitate adaptation
  and problem solving to meet community
  needs
‡Coping, Defensive
  The patient projects falsely positive self-
  evaluation to defend against perceived
  threats to self-esteem
‡Coping, Compromised Family
  Behaviors of significant person to block the
  ability to adapt to the health challenge
‡Coping, Disabled Family
  Behaviors of significant person to block the
  ability to adapt to the health challenge
‡Coping, Readiness for Enhanced Family
  Effective management of adaptive tasks by
  family members involved in patient care
Denial, Ineffective
Dentition, Impaired
Development, Risk for Delayed
Diarrhea
‡Disuse Syndrome, Risk for
  Due to complications of immobility
Diversional Activity, Deficient
Dysreflexia, Autonomic

163

‡Dysreflexia, Autonomic, Risk for
Uninhibited sympathetic response of the nervous system to stressor with a spinal cord injury above T7

‡Energy Field, Disturbed
Disrupted flow of energy around the individual with disharmony of body, mind, or spirit

‡Environmental Interpretation Syndrome, Impaired
Lack of orientation to person, place, and time over more than 3 to 6 months

Failure to Thrive, Adult

*Falls, Risk for

Family Processes, Dysfunctional: Alcoholism

Family Processes, Interrupted

‡Fatigue
Sense of exhaustion

‡Fear
Response to a recognized and realistic danger

Fluid Volume, Deficient

Fluid Volume, Excess

Fluid Volume, Risk for Deficient

Fluid Volume, Imbalanced, Risk for

‡Gas Exchange, Impaired
Oxygenation impaired at the alveolar-capillary membrane

‡Grieving, Anticipatory
Emotional responses to potential loss

‡Grieving, Dysfunctional
Unsuccessful responses at working through the process of loss

‡Growth and Development, Delayed
Delayed norms for his or her age

‡Growth, Risk for Disproportionate
At risk for deviations in norms for his or her age

‡Health Maintenance, Ineffective
Inability to maintain health

‡Health-Seeking Behaviors (Specify)
Person is trying to alter habits to move toward a higher level of health

‡Home Maintenance, Impaired
Inability to maintaining safe home environment

Hopelessness

Hyperthermia

Hypothermia

Identity, Disturbed Personal

Incontinence, Functional Urinary

Incontinence, Reflex Urinary

Incontinence, Stress Urinary

Incontinence, Total Urinary

Incontinence, Urge Urinary

Incontinence, Risk for Urge Urinary

Infant Behavior, Disorganized

Infant Behavior, Risk for Disorganized

Infant Behavior, Readiness for Enhanced Organized

Infant Feeding Pattern, Ineffective

Infection, Risk for

‡Injury, Risk for
Environment interacts negatively with patient's ability to adapt

Injury, Risk for Perioperative-Positioning

‡Intracranial Adaptive Capacity, Decreased
The individual is experiencing increased intracranial pressure

Knowledge, Deficient (Specify)

Loneliness, Risk for

Memory, Impaired

Mobility, Impaired Bed

Mobility, Impaired Physical

Mobility, Impaired Wheelchair

Nausea

Neglect, Unilateral

‡Neurovascular, Peripheral Dysfunction, Risk for
Risk for experiencing lack of circulation, sensation, or motion in an extremity

‡Noncompliance
Failure to adhere to an agreed upon therapeutic plan

‡Nutrition, Imbalanced, Less Than Body Requirements
Insufficient intake of nutrients

‡Nutrition, Imbalanced, More Than Body Requirements
Excess intake of nutrients

Nutrition, Imbalanced, Risk for More Than Body Requirements

Oral Mucous Membrane, Impaired

Pain, Acute

Pain, Chronic

Parenting, Impaired

Parenting, Risk for Impaired

Peripheral Neurovascular Dysfunction, Risk for

Poisoning, Risk for

‡Post-Trauma Syndrome
Maladaptive response to trauma

Post-Trauma Syndrome, Risk for
Powerlessness
*Powerlessness, Risk for
‡Protection, Ineffective
    Inability to protect self from internal or
    external threats to illness or injury such as
    with abnormal blood profiles or
    immunodeficiency
Rape-Trauma Syndrome
Rape-Trauma Syndrome: Compound Reaction
Rape-Trauma Syndrome: Silent Reaction
‡Relocation Stress Syndrome
    Disturbances resulting from transfer from one
    environment to another
*Relocation Stress Syndrome, Risk for
Role Performance, Ineffective
Self-Care Deficit, Bathing/Hygiene
Self-Care Deficit, Dressing/Grooming
Self-Care Deficit, Feeding
Self-Care Deficit, Toileting
Self-Esteem, Chronic Low
Self-Esteem, Situational Low
*Self-Esteem, Risk for Situational Low
*Self-Mutilation
Self-Mutilation, Risk for
‡Sensory Perception, Disturbed (Specify: Visual,
    Auditory, Kinesthetic, Gustatory, Tactile,
    Olfactory)
    Altered sensory perceptions with impaired
    response to stimuli
‡Sexual Dysfunction
    Patient is experiencing a change in sexual
    function perceived as unsatisfying
‡Sexuality Patterns, Ineffective
    Patient expresses concern about sexuality
Skin Integrity, Impaired
Skin Integrity, Risk for Impaired
Sleep Deprivation
Sleep Pattern, Disturbed
‡Social Interaction, Impaired
    Insufficient, excessive, ineffective social
    exchanges
Social Isolation
‡Sorrow, Chronic
    Sorrow in response to continued loss such as
    throughout the trajectory of an illness
‡Spiritual Distress
    Disruption in life principles that transcend
    nature

Spiritual Distress, Risk for
‡Spiritual Well-Being, Readiness for Enhanced
    Inner strength and harmony with self, others,
    and higher power and the environment
Suffocation, Risk for
*Suicide, Risk for
Surgical Recovery, Delayed
Swallowing, Impaired
Therapeutic Regimen: Effective Management
‡Therapeutic Regimen: Ineffective Management
    Inability to integrate a treatment program
    into daily living
Therapeutic Regimen: Community, Ineffective
    Management
Therapeutic Regimen: Family, Ineffective
    Management
Thermoregulation, Ineffective
‡Thought Process, Disturbed
    Disrupted cognition
‡Tissue Integrity, Impaired
    Altered body tissues due to any cause
‡Tissue Perfusion, Ineffective (Specify Type:
    Renal, Cerebral, Cardiopulmonary,
    Gastrointestinal, Peripheral)
    Decreased tissue perfusion at capillary level
Transfer Ability, Impaired
Trauma, Risk for
Urinary Elimination, Impaired
Urinary Retention
Ventilation, Impaired Spontaneous
Ventilatory Weaning Response, Dysfunctional
Violence, Risk for Other-Directed
Violence, Risk for Self-Directed
Walking, Impaired
*Wandering

---

*New to the 14th Conference
†Permission from North American Nursing Diagnosis
Association (2001). NANDA Nursing Diagnoses:
Definitions and Classification, 2001–2002. Philadelphia:
NANDA. Copyright 2001, by the North American
Nursing Diagnosis Association.
‡Definitions are added for clarification of those
diagnoses that are not self-explanatory.
**Please also see the NANDA diagnoses grouped
according to Gordon's Functional Health Patterns.**

# Index